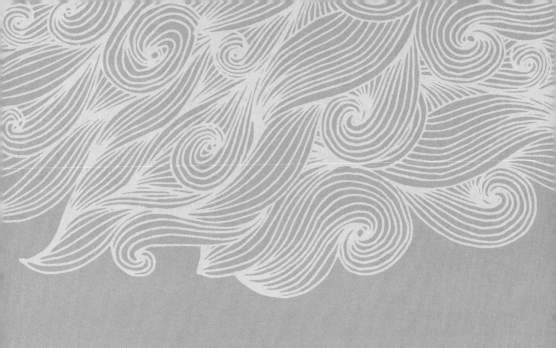

THE POWER OF
GUIDED MEDITATION

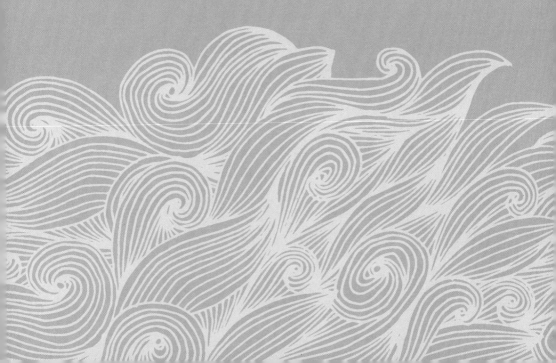

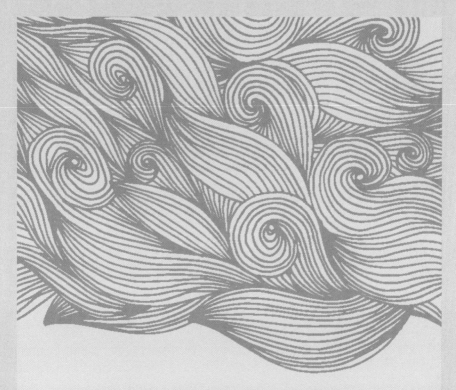

THE POWER OF
GUIDED MEDITATION

SIMPLE PRACTICES TO PROMOTE WELLBEING

JESSICA CROW

FAIR WINDS

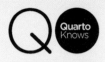

Inspiring | Educating | Creating | Entertaining

Brimming with creative inspiration, how-to projects, and useful
information to enrich your everyday life, Quarto Knows is a favorite
destination for those pursuing their interests and passions. Visit our
site and dig deeper with our books into your area of interest:
Quarto Creates, Quarto Cooks, Quarto Homes, Quarto Lives,
Quarto Drives, Quarto Explores, Quarto Gifts, or Quarto Kids.

25 24 23 22 21 1 2 3 4 5

ISBN: 978-1-58923-989-0

Digital edition published in 2021

QUAR.340577

Conceived, edited, and designed by Quarto Publishing plc.
6 Blundell Street, London N7 9BH

Senior Commissioning Editor: Eszter Karpati
Editor: Caroline West
Art Director: Gemma Wilson
Designer: Karin Skånberg
Junior Designer: India Minter
Publisher: Samantha Warrington

Printed in Singapore

The information in this book is for educational purposes
only. It is not intended to replace the advice of a physician or
medical practitioner. Please see your health-care provider
before beginning any new health program.

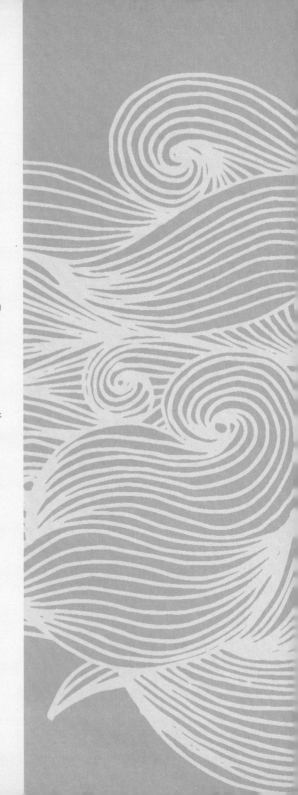

Contents

Meet Jessica 6

About This Book 8

Creating the Journey 12

Preparing for Meditation 14

CHAPTER 1 MINDFUL 16

MINDFULNESS MEDITATIONS 18
1. Body Scan 20
2. Mindful Awareness of the Breath 26
3. Mindful Awareness of Sounds 32
4. Mindful Awareness of Thoughts 38
5. Mindful Eating 44
6. Mindfulness of Support
   from the Ground 46
7. Mindfulness of Walking 48
8. Mindfulness of Compassion 50
9. Mindful Listening
   & Communication 54

CHAPTER 2 CALM 58

FINDING CALM 60
10. Calming Breath 62
11. Stress Reduction SSS-Breath 68
12. Breathing for Physical Release 70
13. Progressive Muscle Relaxation 72

14. Affirming Serenity 75
15. Ocean Breath 78
16. Belly Breathing 80
17. Countdown to Sleep 85
18. Easy Sleep 87
19. Guided Sleep Relaxation 89

CHAPTER 3 VISUALIZE 92

VISUALIZATION 94
20. Energy Boost 96
21. Dissolve Mental Stress 98
22. Heart Health 100
23. Immunity Boost 103
24. Releasing Negativity 106
25. Freeing Sadness & Grief 108
26. Wake Up with Confidence 110
27. Wake Up to Radiant Health 113
28. Calming Color Therapy 115
29. Accessing Your Inner Genius 117
30. Yoga Nidra Deep
    Healing Relaxation 119

Meditation Directory 122

Index 127

Acknowledgments 128

Recorded Guided Meditations 128

Meet Jessica

A decade ago I was at the end of a long-term partnership and suddenly in the midst of a big medical scare. I had no stress-management tools. I knew that if I wanted to feel better each day and live with purpose, I needed to change my lifestyle to include tools for anxiety reduction and mindful ways to reconnect to my higher self.

It was during this time that I was guided to yoga and meditation. I gradually built up my daily practices and studies before attending my first teacher training. It wasn't long before I began to sense changes in my physical and mental states. As I started to feel better and regain personal power, I became fascinated with the brain and the power of thought.

I went back to school in order to study neurobiology and psychology in-depth. My future plan was drawn up—or so I thought. I planned to finish my Bachelor of Science and segue into a program at Stanford University to study the neural correlates of compassion, fear, and intuition as they related to modern social behavior. Right around the time I finished my degree and was seeking out internships, I happened to meet my yoga teacher, the world-renowned Sri Dharma Mittra.

Sri Dharma Mittra imparted to me the importance of developing the intuition to guide you on your path and the daily practice of genuine compassion. Both of these were synchronistically in-line with my scientific enthusiasm and I ended up creating a new intuitive path—teaching the science of yoga. Now, after years

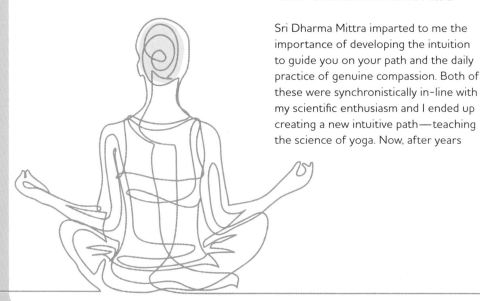

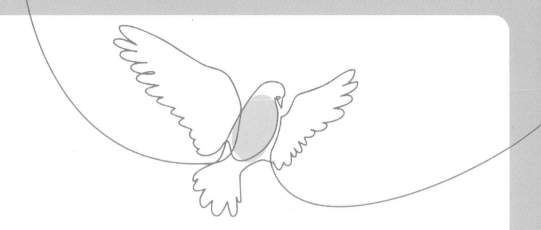

You already have everything you need
to heal yourself and to live your life
with purpose, passion, and joy.
Reconnect... again and again.
All is within.

and years of practice, additional study, investigation, and integration, I've learned to weave this knowledge into my everyday life. It's made a world of difference. I've learned how to stand up for my intuitive sense and nurture my own health through yoga, meditation, and mindfulness.

I am grateful that I can now help guide other people in their quest for healing and a bigger sense of connection in their lives. It gives me joy to share these methods with others and to see them rediscover and trust their own innate ability to reinvent their lives and expand beyond what they thought was possible.

My intention in writing this book is to provide the reader with an easy and accessible way to meditate, to help them reduce stress, connect with their higher self, and live mindfully, building a better relationship with themselves and other people in their lives. Meditation is a practice that anyone can learn and the benefits are far-reaching. As you build up your meditation practice and gain experience, you will find that these benefits extend into every area of your life.

About This Book

The book is organized into three main chapters that invite you into a relationship with your body and mind through a nonjudgmental lens.

CHAPTER 1
MINDFUL
pages 16–57

This chapter explores how mindfulness practices can help bring your attention to the present moment. Place the attention on how the body and breath feel and also what thoughts and emotions are present. Learn key mindfulness techniques, including a body scan and breath awareness.

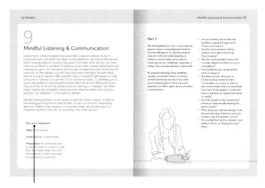

States whether a meditation has one, two, or three parts. For longer meditations, you can do just one or two parts, or all three. However, it is recommended that you work through the parts chronologically.

FEATURED MEDITATIONS

1. Body scan
Learn to *rest your attention* on the ever-changing sensations in your physical body.

2. Mindful Awareness of the Breath
Learn how to use the breath as a *present-moment anchor.*

3. Mindful Awareness of Sounds
Practice observing your mind's *reaction to sounds* with detachment.

4. Mindful Awareness of Thoughts
Practice observing your *thoughts without judgment* and with acceptance.

5. Mindful Eating
Connect with your relationship to the food you eat at a *deeper level.*

6. Mindfulness of Support from the Ground
Explore the unique awareness of sensations and flexibility that a *standing position* provides.

7. Mindfulness of Walking
Use shifting sensations in your body and surroundings as tools for strengthening *present-moment* awareness while walking.

8. Mindfulness of Compassion
Use meditation to *send loving-kindness* to others while expanding your own capacity for love and compassion.

9. Mindful Listening & Communication
Learn how to communicate *fully and be authentically present* in everyday communication.

CHAPTER 2
CALM

pages 58–91

Learn how to employ specific techniques to induce a feeling of calm and relaxation, and so lead a more stress-free life. Use the meditations in this section to release physical tension, reduce anxiety, and ensure a good night's sleep.

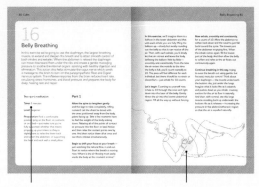

States how long a meditation takes to practice and also whether it is suitable for a beginner or someone with more experience.

Shading, where relevant, will show where to focus your attention during a meditation.

10. Calming Breath
Count and equalize your inhales and exhales to induce a state of *calm relaxation*.

11. Stress Reduction SSS-Breath
Relax quickly with this technique, by making the exhale longer than the inhale.

12. Breathing for Physical Release
Combine *controlled breathing* with visualization for a powerful healing effect.

13. Progressive Muscle Relaxation
Induce a feeling of complete relaxation by *tensing and releasing* all parts of the body.

14. Affirming Serenity
Learn how to use *positive affirmations* to improve self-confidence and self-esteem.

15. Ocean Breath
Add sounds to inhales and exhales to create a *meditative focus* in this calming breathing exercise.

16. Belly Breathing
Practice controlled *diaphragmatic breathing* to calm the nervous system for overall health.

17. Countdown to Sleep
Learn how counting can be used to settle thoughts and calm emotions, to ensure a *good night's sleep*.

18. Easy Sleep
Fall into a deep and *restorative sleep* quickly and easily.

19. Guided Sleep Relaxation
Release as much *physical tension* and stress as possible to achieve deeper sleep.

»

CHAPTER 3
VISUALIZE
pages 92–121

Discover how using visualization techniques during meditation can emphasize the healing process with intentionality. The exercises in this section address things like recurring thought patterns, physical health and energy levels, and self-confidence.

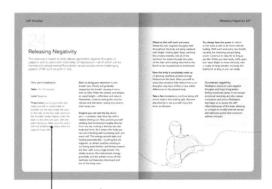

Suggests the best position to adopt for the meditation and also gives advice, if necessary, on anything else you need to do before starting.

20. Energy Boost
Refresh and recharge *body, mind, and spirit* in a few short minutes.

21. Dissolve Mental Stress
Relieve *headaches* and begin to release unhealthy thought patterns.

22. Heart Health
Restore and *heal your heart* both physically and emotionally.

23. Immunity Boost
Strengthen your immune system for *improved health* and wellbeing.

24. Releasing Negativity
Start to shift negative mental fluctuations into *positivity and resilience*.

25. Freeing Sadness & Grief
Release the *grip of negative feelings* that may be suppressed and trapped in the body.

26. Wake Up with Confidence
A helpful exercise to *boost confidence and positivity* as you begin your day.

27. Wake Up to Radiant Health
Start a *new day* full of health, energy, and vitality.

28. Calming Color Therapy
Relax and heal your mind and body with the *power of color*.

29. Accessing Your Inner Genius
A meditation to help *stimulate and inspire* your unique gifts, passions, and creativity.

30. Yoga Nidra Deep Healing Relaxation
Access a state between sleep and wakefulness to direct your *inner life force* to promote healing.

MEDITATION DIRECTORY
pages 122–126

This section recommends the most suitable meditations to alleviate the symptoms of some common conditions, including insomnia, chronic pain, and depression.

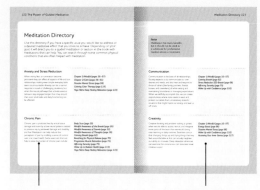

Gives an overview of a range of common conditions that can be alleviated through regular meditation.

Gives suggestions for the best meditations to use for specific conditions and ailments.

Important note

Before you begin, make sure to read the key information and tips on *Preparing for Meditation* (pages 14–15).

"It helps to remember that our practice is not about accomplishing anything—not about winning or losing—but about ceasing to struggle and relaxing as it is. That is what we are doing when we sit down to meditate. That attitude spreads into the rest of our lives."

Pema Chödrön

Creating the Journey

Starting a meditation practice takes curiosity, but making it a regular part of your routine calls for a desire for change and self-empowerment. It also requires consistency and dedication—even if that means sparing just 5–10 minutes a day in the beginning. On the surface, the meditation practices may seem extremely simple and easy. However, when we place all our attention within each exercise we become aware of the subtle complexities and personal challenges that present themselves. But these are normal stepping stones to growth and the "enlightening" of the conscious mind by observing and perhaps challenging the subconscious.

Over time, the basic tools and exercises involved in meditation become second nature, and we gradually learn to extend the benefits of meditation and mindfulness into any given moment of our lives. We learn to recognize the true quality of our thoughts as they arise.

With this information we become more and more aware of the usefulness or negative effects of our ongoing internal dialogues. With practice, we also become skilled at making a determination more and more quickly: right after the thoughts occur, while the thoughts are taking place, and sometimes (ideally) before they even take hold.

Using the power of this awareness we can then disregard or switch the thoughts to something more beneficial before they have a physiological effect on our health, or continue to fuel an undesirable mental pattern that we're keen to dislodge.

Benefits of meditation

Many studies have been conducted, particularly over the last decade, and these suggest that regular meditation is strongly associated with positive effects on decision-making and self-control, increases in productivity and focus, better physical health, and a decreased perception of pain. It can also help reduce stress and improve all our human relationships and interactions.

As you develop a consistent practice, you'll notice that these exercises strengthen your concentration and increase your sensitivity to the state of your health and all thoughts related to it at every level— physical, mental, emotional, and spiritual.

Working with internal dialogues

It is a little counterintuitive that something as basic as meditation could be seen as so challenging for many of us to integrate into our lives. But the nature of the mind is to follow thoughts, to create stories and fantasies, to play into "what-ifs" and "could-haves," and basically to stay as active as possible switching between these during our waking hours. The mind is also used to perpetuating stories of who we are—what we look and feel like, what we are capable of, as well as all the myriad qualities that separate "us" from "other."

Such internal dialogues are constantly circling in the background of our subconscious mind—some originating from early memories and associations, the opinions of others, and cultural and societal expectations. Yet many of them are more consciously chosen and re-chosen by us alone, daily, hourly, and in every moment. That is why we all have significant power to change ourselves, and the power is in this moment, in the choices we are making right now.

We suddenly see clear connections between body, breath, and thoughts—cause-and-effect relationships that, to a large extent, determine our mood, energy and motivation, physical health, and general sense of how we believe our life is unfolding. Sometimes when we start a meditation practice, we may come head-to-head with internal challenges and restrictions as the light of our awareness becomes more focused and refined. At such times, we are witnessing the mindscape and being given a chance to begin a little design work on our thoughts and intentions.

A child's inner wisdom

Children have a natural propensity for meditation. They can become so completely absorbed in whatever they are doing, seeing, or hearing that nothing else can break their "attentional" force field. Since children are naturally curious about how and why things work, they hone in on things with their full attention (and, even if that attention doesn't last long, it is uniquely one-pointed and direct).

It is this same sense of curiosity that we are trying to cultivate and maintain as we begin self-study practices like meditation. We can use meditation to gaze inward and act like an interested observer—to enlist our own "inner scientist" to watch and take mental notes, so that, over time, we make connections and come to rational, yet intuitive, conclusions about our state of being and what we really need to do for ourselves to shift our life experience.

Preparing for Meditation

While some types of meditation practice suggest that you sit straight up, others may require you to walk or lie down. As we move through the various practices in the book, the suggested posture for each is given at the start of the exercise. In general, though, the spine should be kept as straight and long as possible. There are two reasons for this:

Firstly, in Eastern philosophy and medicine, the spine is said to be the approximate location of the chakras, the seven or more energy centers that control and respond to different aspects of our being and are always trying to find homeostasis, or to rebalance themselves. The spinal canal also houses the main channel of energy, or vital life force, and two additional smaller channels related to the breath. Some types of meditation are said to release blockages to this energy so that it can easily flow up and down the spinal canal, so increasing vital health.

Secondly, when the spine is lifted or lengthened, the force of the supporting musculature becomes more evenly balanced—or, ideally, it becomes close to neutral (as is seen when you apply a plumb line). When the ears are moved over the shoulders, the shoulders are brought over the hips, and the hips are aligned over the ankles, the mechanical force exerted by the postural muscles is kept to a minimum. In general, this results in less muscular pain and fatigue when you are sitting for meditation. This position also allows the breath to be more full, anatomically creating space for the lungs and smaller breathing muscles to expand more, and for the diaphragm to stretch deeper into the abdomen, bringing more air in with each breath.

Many people work hunched over a computer, desk, or mobile device. For this reason, finding alignment in the spine can prove difficult. This is because there is already a muscular imbalance in the body, with some muscles tighter and weaker than they should be, and the opposing muscles overstretched and weak. As a result, it can feel uncomfortable or strenuous for some people to even sit up straight in the beginning. If this happens and it distracts you from the practice, simply begin seated against a wall, so that your back and the back of your head can gently rest against it when needed. Over time, the muscles needed to remain upright for longer periods will strengthen and the body will find a more efficient method of remaining there, allowing you to focus more on the meditation session.

Some people prefer to set the tone of their day with early or mid-morning meditation, while others like to practice at night when their work for the day is done. As a general rule for beginners, choose a time and stick with it for a while. Set up a reminder in your calendar and be consistent about the length of the practice—starting at five minutes and increasing by increments of five minutes every few weeks or so. Think of your meditation time as self-care for your mind and spirit—just as you set aside time to brush your teeth or take a shower, firmly commit to a few minutes of reconnection each day.

Tips for Getting Started

It's beneficial to read through the meditation that you're preparing to practice at least once or twice before engaging in the exercise. This will give you context and allow you to keep more of your focus internally. It's highly recommended that you use a voice recorder (most smartphones have this feature) to record yourself reading the exercise, so that you can simply play it back and follow the directions and dialogue without moving too much or opening your eyes. You could also have a friend or family member read it out to you.

- Most of the meditations take between 5 and 20 minutes. If you are a beginner, you may want to start with a shorter time and then extend the practice as you gain more experience.
- If you wish, you can use a timer when meditating, but this isn't necessary unless stated in the Preparation notes.
- You can meditate sitting on a chair or on the floor, or lying on your back. Experiment to see what works best for you and then choose a position that feels the most comfortable from those recommended for each exercise.
- When meditating on the floor, you may want to use a cushion, pillow, or yoga mat, to ensure you are as comfortable as possible.

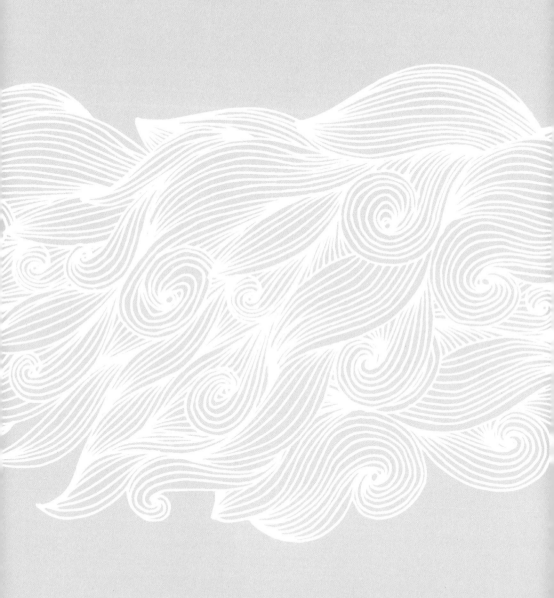

CHAPTER 1
MINDFUL

Mindfulness is the practice of bringing one's focus back to the present, back to the here and now. Our attention becomes centered on this moment—how the body feels, how the breath feels, what emotions are active, or what types of thoughts are entering and exiting the mind.

Mindfulness Meditations

Although there is some overlap, mindfulness is not only meditation and meditation is not only mindfulness. Mindfulness in its most complete sense is a way of living, thinking, and being that is self-aware and deliberate.

Most mindfulness meditation practices, as we know them in the West, are rooted in Buddhism, but the idea of mindfulness has been an essential part of numerous cultures and religions throughout history.

Research has shown that consistent mindfulness meditation practice contributes to the construction, growth, and connectivity of certain brain networks that govern self-control and emotional regulation. Building and strengthening neural networks in these regions can help practitioners build virtues such as patience and insight that can then be extended into everyday life.

Neural circuitry that stores and produces self-referential information (our own collection of stories that we hold about ourselves and what we deeply believe to be true about our life experiences) is altered and transformed during meditation practices. It becomes more malleable and easily influenced by new thoughts. This gives us a perfect opportunity to reconstruct the architecture of our brains in order to determine who we actually believe we are in this world, what we think we can accomplish, and what we think we deserve and allow ourselves to have. Meditation also seems to improve the overall experience of one's everyday life.

When our entire focus is devoted to the present moment, the brain naturally lets go of ruminations about the past and the future.

When our entire focus is devoted to the present moment, the brain naturally lets go of ruminations about the past and the future. All of our mental energy goes toward becoming as sensitive as possible to how we feel right now. As we inquire and become familiar with how the body feels, how the breath acts, and how the thoughts present themselves at different points in time, we start to realize that they're all intimately connected.

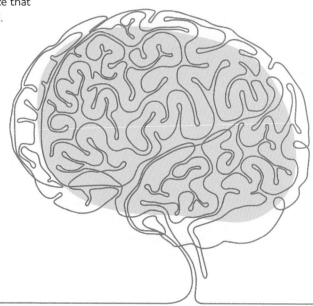

1

Body Scan

During the body scan exercises we learn to consciously direct our attention to our physical body parts, one by one. We learn simply to take notice of what sensations and feelings may be presenting themselves at any point in time, and we practice allowing them to be as they are—without trying to change them, knowing that they will shift and change depending on many factors, from moment to moment, or day to day. In this way, we can begin to realize the depth of the connection between our body and mindstate.

Two-part meditation

Takes 5–20 minutes

Level Beginner to Intermediate

Preparation Find any comfortable seated position on a chair or a cushion on the floor.

Part 1

Sit comfortably and allow your seat to really heavy-down, grounding into the chair or cushion. At the same time, encourage your spine to lengthen upward, lifting your head effortlessly toward the ceiling. Resting your arms and hands where they feel most comfortable, allow your eyes to close softly. Just notice the sensation of your natural breath now for a moment...

Imagine your mental attention is like a concentrated beam of light, like a flashlight. Slowly bring this beam of attention down to your feet. Feel your feet and their placement on the floor or cushion. And, with a sense of curiosity and soft awareness, just notice any sensations, physical or otherwise, at the level of your feet and toes. Notice the pressure of the feet resting on the floor or touching the body, the seat, or your shoes. Notice if there is any sense of vibration or pulsing, any feeling of temperature or pressure, stillness or energy, or anything else that you can pinpoint about how the feet feel at this moment in time. Simply notice any sensations that may be present right now in the feet, without moving them. If you can't make out any particular sensations at this point in time, that's fine too. Just notice that and move to the next area.

Now leave the feet be, and gently move your attention to the lower legs. Take notice of anything that arises there— any sensation and movement, any sense of restriction or space. With an alert attention, observe any feeling at all that may arise in the lower legs. Are the sensations the same on each side, or are they different?

And bringing your attention now to the knees—as if you could look all the way inside, noticing any feeling or sensation that presents itself around the knees.

And slowly gliding your attention over the upper legs and thighs, noticing any points of pressure and points of contact... noticing any sensation of weight, heaviness, or lightness. Also notice any feelings or emotions that may be presenting themselves when your full attention is placed on each body part.

Bring your attention up to the hips and the seat now, feeling into the general area without trying to change anything. Just notice what is present right now at the hips and the seat.

Move the focus now to the abdomen— what do you notice when you gaze internally around the area of the abdomen? Practice being accepting of whatever arises. Even if nothing arises right away—that's fine, too.

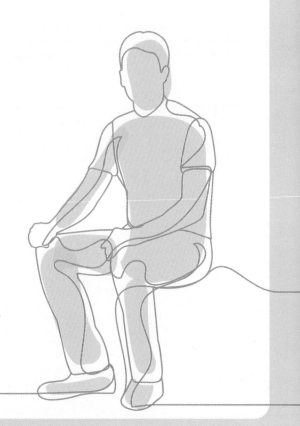

Now move your attention up even further into the rib cage and the chest. Keep observing any and all sensations—any sense of fullness, lightness, expansiveness, limitation, movement, or vibration. Try to remain the observer, not getting involved and yet noticing any feeling at all that may come in or drift off again.

Now bring your attention to the lower back—the lower spine and the muscles around it. What can you observe at the level of the lower back? How does it feel right now? Keep witnessing the body as it is, letting any desire to judge or criticize fade away. Right now, you're only an observer, just watching what's already there and remaining unconcerned.

Now bring your attention up to the middle back—the middle spine and the muscles around it. Slowly and gently scanning the area for information… noticing… with a soft, inward gaze.

Move all the way up to the upper back and shoulder blade area. Witnessing any sensation that comes to mind as you rest your focus on the upper back, then on the upper arms, elbows, and forearms. Notice any softness or tightness, any coolness or warmth. Anything that appears in the arms.

And then placing your attention at the hands and fingers. Notice the position of the hands and fingers without any need to change anything.

Bring your attention up to the neck and throat, and just observe with your attention. Just watch this area and stay receptive to what can be found here. Try not to judge in any way, even if a sensation is uncomfortable.

Move your focus to the face now. See the jaw and all the tiny muscles that create the facial expressions. Notice the shape and the feeling of the entire face and witness any emotions or feeling-states that may reside here. Remember, just watching.

And now bring your attention to the top of the head, noticing anything that may stand out. What can you sense around the head and the top of the skull?

Now draw your entire awareness outward, increasing the size of its beam so it can witness the entire body. And notice any sensations, feelings, and moods of the body as a whole. Just noticing very lightly, without needing to attach labels such as "like" or "dislike" to anything that may arise. See if you can remain neutral to the expression of the body as it is, right now.

And now slowly draw your attention back in so that it rests in the very center of the chest, and notice here the rising and falling motion that is always happening.

Begin to breathe a little deeper now, bringing yourself back into the feeling of the body resting in the seat.

Then, when you're ready, softly open your eyes and bring your inner awareness back into the room. Take a moment to notice how you feel right now.

that occurs to you while you hone in on this body part.

Now very gently move your focus up to the ankles and lower legs, as if you're guiding a flashlight to shine your attention on each area. Notice any sensation here without becoming involved in *why* the sensation is occurring or *what* it means—just continue observing it. Practice receiving, welcoming any type of information with open, soft awareness.

Part 2

Begin by positioning yourself comfortably and allow your body to relax down into the support of the seat. Let your spine lift up and lengthen, as the shoulders rest down and back. Leave the arms wherever they're most comfortable, with the palms up or down on the lap. Just begin by closing your eyes softly.

Start to move your attention down to the feet now. Fully place your awareness at the feet. Notice here any sensation that makes itself known. Do you sense the pressure of the feet where they meet the floor, or perhaps where they touch your shoes... Take note of any other sensation

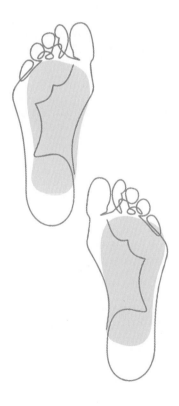

Now guiding your attention up to the knees. And gently gaze inside, as if you have X-ray vision, and notice what's taking place there.

Attending to the upper legs and thighs now, notice any sense of weight, vibration, pulsating—any physical sensation at all, but also any feeling or sense of emotion that may be in the vicinity.

Now guide your pure attention up to the hips, the seat, and the pelvic area. As if you can gaze all the way inside and take mental notes on what's occurring there in this moment. Try to maintain a sense of curiosity about what you may find.

Move your attention to the abdomen, sensing any movement, any energy, any feeling-state at all—without concern.

Bring your attention now up to the chest and rib cage, and see what presents itself there. What kind of movement occurs, and what does that movement *feel* like right now? What type of message may be present if you tune in a little more deeply? Without trying to interpret anything that comes up, simply notice it for what it is.

Now to the lower back, feeling into this area with an attitude of self-discovery—a bit like a scientist, observing layer by layer...

Guiding the focus to the middle back now. Enhance your sensitivity and take notice. Can you observe your posture without shifting it?

And to the upper back and shoulder blade area. With your open awareness turned in on this area, simply remain present with whatever turns up.

Bring your attention to the shoulders now. Observing their placement in space. Looking into and through.

And to the upper arms, then the elbows and forearms. What sensations exist in the arms right now? Does placing your attention there make you want to move, or become more still?

Now move your attention to the wrists and hands, and slowly shine the light of your attention all the way down to the fingertips. Notice what conditions and qualities are present.

Focus now on the neck and throat area. Notice what this area feels like, while releasing any desire to judge or to follow any thought about why any particular sensation has arisen. Just remain present with what is there, right now.

Noticing the jaw and face. Notice the shape, the expression. What does it feel like? Is there tension? Is there softness? Notice only what is there right now.

And, finally, move your attention up to the top of the head. Staying curious. Staying neutral as you observe and sense the scalp and the top of the skull.

And now gently begin to expand your sphere of attention so that it takes in the shape of the entire body as it exists right now. Notice if there is any overlying feeling or sensation in the landscape of the physical body in this moment. Be sensitive. And be open. And if nothing presents itself, remain unconcerned.

Now very gently bring your awareness to the center of the chest once again. Notice the rising and falling motion that is continually happening there as the breath enters and exits the body. Notice this breath begin to deepen slightly, as you feel your body again on your seat, and your presence slowly comes back into the room.

Slowly open your eyes. And notice how you feel right now, in this moment.

Acceptance

The body scan technique is a wonderful tool for cultivating concentration and the conscious direction of mental attention, but it also helps us to accept some things that we may find challenging about our physical being. Often, once we learn to accept something, it may begin to change, shift, or heal on its own.

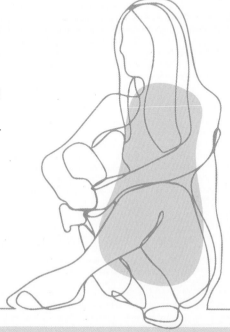

2

Mindful Awareness of the Breath

The breath is used as an anchor or a guiding post in many types of meditation because of its constant, automatic nature. It's a physical focal point that is always happening—all by itself. When we become mindful of the qualities of the breath we gain information about current thoughts, feelings, and emotions and how they influence the breath, and vice versa.

Three-part meditation

Takes 5–20 minutes

Level Beginner to Intermediate

Preparation Find any comfortable seated position on a chair or a cushion on the floor.

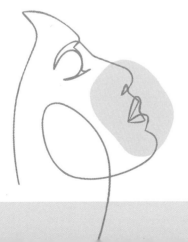

Part 1

Find a comfortable seated position where the spine can be long and straight, either sitting in a chair or on the floor. You can also lie on your back if you wish. Soften the shoulders and relax the eyelids to a softly closed position.

Begin now by feeling your breath. Notice how the breath feels right now to you, without trying to change anything. Now notice its qualities: does it feel deep or shallow? Warm or cool? Energized or relaxed? Restricted or expansive?

Just notice the breath's natural rhythm, and notice any movement or motion in the body that comes with it.

If at any time you notice your mind being drawn away by thoughts, simply acknowledge that the mind has wandered and bring your attention right back to the sensations of the breath. Keep returning to the feeling of it moving in and out of the body right now.

Notice if the breath is moving fully, and if it's moving into every available area. Does the breath make its way into the lower abdomen, or not? Can you sense it in the lower back? And does it expand into the side-body? Try not to judge anything that you witness. There is no right or wrong; there is only how it feels right *now*.

Take a moment now to notice where you're sensing the movement of the air entering and exiting the body the most. Is there one point or are there multiple places? If you are quiet, and alert, can you feel the airflow at the tips of the nostrils, the back of the throat, the chest, back, belly? All of them?

Each time thoughts distract your attention, recognize that the mind is simply being drawn away (which is its nature) and then gently turn your awareness back to the movement and sensations of the breath.

Practice trying not to judge anything that you may notice arising with the breath. For a few minutes, be the observer of its activity. Watch curiously, with a desire to become familiar with how your breath and energy move—right now in this present moment.

Your only task right now is to be with the breath. To travel in and out of the body riding this wave—in and out, again and again. And simply to notice what is taking place and what the activity of the breath feels like. This automatic movement that is always happening—whether we're conscious of it or not—is providing us with an essential life-giving force.

Sometimes the breath changes or shifts just by bringing our awareness toward it. Just by shining our full attention onto it—onto the intricacies and details of this constant motion. Become aware if any qualities of your breath have shifted as you focus your attention in on them.

Without concern, still watching. There is no sense of judgment, no condemnation. No right or wrong. Just getting to know how the breath behaves and responds to the body.

And when you're ready, slowly begin to bring your awareness back to the whole body—noticing the body in its seat or lying down. Feeling the weight of the body, the air on the skin and face.

And very slowly... allow your eyes to open. Take a moment to notice how you feel right now.

Part 2

Find a comfortable seated position and let your back be as straight and long as possible, with as little effort as possible. Notice the outermost muscles of the body, especially on the front of the body, begin to soften. Feel comfortable. And then gently close your eyes.

Bring your attention to the sensation of your breath—as it exists right now, without trying to change it. Focus your attention on how the breath feels at this point in time. Allow the breath to be completely natural, with its own rhythm. And allow the body to move slightly as it will, responding to the in- and out-breath waves. Notice those areas of the body that move the most as you breathe. And also notice any areas of the body where you feel the air may not be reaching completely—areas that may feel closed off or restricted.

Notice the areas of the body where you feel the most sensation from the breath now. That may be an aura of warmth or coolness, the feeling of air brushing the skin or traveling internally, the rising and falling at the center of the chest. Maybe you notice the spreading and lifting of the rib cage, or movement within the belly. In which places do you feel the presence of the breath the most strongly, right now in this moment?

What other qualities can you pinpoint on the breath? If you were a scientist watching this breath for the *very* first time, what would be most notable, most obvious? What could you learn by witnessing your breath anew?

Continue to leave your full attention on the breath—trying to cultivate a sense of curiosity. Just simple, easy, childlike curiosity. Leave out all sense of expectation or judgment of how the breath should, would, or could feel.

If you notice your mind has wandered, or if you feel the thoughts begin to pull you away, gently notice where you've gone and then kindly guide your attention back. Rest your awareness on the breath. The breath is now serving as your anchor. When thoughts come in and attempt to distract or disturb the steadiness of your focus, just keep coming back again and again to your anchor. Find stability there on the constant breath.

Continuing to notice the sensation of the breath as it exists in each moment—that constant flow, like waves coming in and then going back out to sea.

Perhaps checking to see if the behavior of the breath has shifted at all as you've concentrated your full awareness onto it, again and again. Is the breath now presenting any new qualities? Or does it feel the same as when you started? There is no right or wrong. Simply noticing.

When you're ready, start to bring your awareness back into the room. Feel your physical body in relation to the room. Let your eyes flutter open softly. And notice how you feel right now.

Part 3

Find a comfortable seated position that helps you stay alert and attentive. The spine should be long and upright, but the rest of the body can be fairly soft and relaxed,

including the face and the eyelids as they drop closed. Begin now by noticing your breath. Just notice it as it is right now.

Feel the rising and falling in the center of the chest. Is this movement large? Is it vibratory? Look at the quality of the air as it touches the tip of the nose at the edges of the nostrils. Notice if the breath feels shallow or expansive right now.

Don't attempt to change the breath. Does it feel static or invigorating? Cool or warm? Notice what feelings and sensations come to you right now as you place your spotlight of attention solely on the breath.

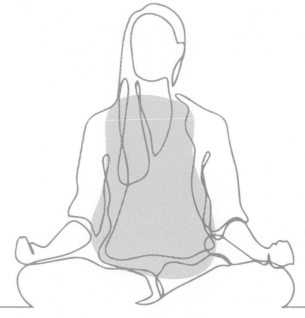

It may help to imagine that you have never witnessed this breath before. And, in fact, every breath is brand new. The inhale that you just took will be slightly different to the one that's about to arrive. Just continue to watch as new sensations or movements might present themselves. Please try not to judge. There is no right or wrong.

Your only task is to observe from an unbiased place, a neutral place. Just inquire gently and learn about how your breath moves and how it engages with your body and mind.

The nature of the mind is to be very active, and so it tends to follow any train of thought that happens to pass by— daydreams and whims, memories, future plans. The mind will try many things to keep it from remaining one-pointed for very long, especially in the beginning. Try anyway. As soon as you notice that the mind has interjected and led you off on some other pathway, just very simply and gently guide your attention back again to the anchor of the breath. Each and every time that your mind wanders and you're able to bring it back to your point of attention, your concentration becomes stronger and stronger. You're building up your mental muscles—literally forging stronger neural networks in the brain that help improve your meditation and power of mind.

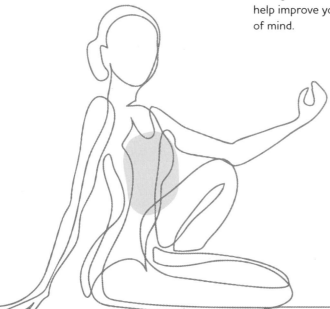

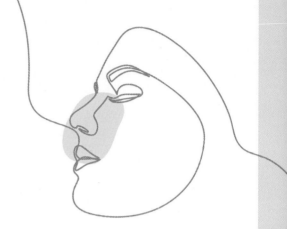

So when a thought comes in again, simply acknowledge it, and then come right back to the breath. Notice any sensation. How the breath is moving, where it's moving, and anything else it may be expressing to you.

Sometimes an emotion or feeling-state may come up in the body as you're attending to the breath. And in the same way that you would with a distracting thought, just notice something has arisen that has borrowed your attention for the moment. And then very gently come back again to the present sensations of the breath.

The only thing that we are interested in right now is the experience of the present, this moment, the Now—the most powerful moment that exists.

Checking in now, observe if there have been any noticeable shifts in the qualities of the breath since you began this exercise.

And when you feel ready, start to bring yourself back to the feeling of your physical body.

Then begin to open your eyes, gently bringing yourself back into the room. Take a moment or two to notice how you feel right now.

The breath as anchor
Returning the awareness to the breath gives us access to the power of the present moment, while helping to loosen rumination and replay of the past, or anxiety and worry about the future. The in- and out-flow of the breath is the epitome of "Now."

3

Mindful Awareness of Sounds

Like thoughts, sounds have a transient nature and can easily pull up very personal emotional associations. These qualities make sounds a perfect focal point for mindfulness exercises because we have many chances to follow the emotional ties and then bring the mind back again, each time strengthening the brain's capacity for one-pointed attention and enhancing our mindful listening skills. Practice patience.

Three-part meditation

Takes 5–20 minutes

Level Beginner to Intermediate

Preparation Find any comfortable seated position on a chair or a cushion on the floor.

Part 1

Find a comfortable seated position, keeping your back tall and erect and resting your arms and legs comfortably. Get the sense that you're well-grounded into your seat, whether this is on a chair or cushion. Feel the spine very softly lifting up, and the back of the neck lengthening.

Allow your eyes to close as you bring your attention inward to the rising and falling of the breath happening right around the center of the chest. Without trying to change the breath at all, just witness this motion—this undulating movement of in and out. Sense the breath fully going in, then sense it fully coming back out. This is your grounding, your anchor, and you can always return to it at any point.

Start to expand your attention now. Watch your field of awareness growing larger until it can take in the entire landscape of the body now. Still holding an awareness of the rhythmic breath, but now feeling it throughout the whole body.

Just allowing the breath to be... exactly as it is right now. A rising and falling. The constant pulse of life feeding the body.

Begin to shift your focus from the body and breath to the sounds in the environment around you. Become aware of the sounds that are nearby, as well as the sounds that are farther away. Imagine you can allow any and all sounds to just come and go—on their own.

There's no need to reach out to find or actively listen to or search for the sounds. Just allow your body to be like a receiver—allow the sounds to come and to go as they will. You are like one big microphone, sitting and breathing there, picking up all of the surrounding vibrational currents. They arise in different forms and frequencies, and then they dissipate again. Even the spaces between sounds, even the silence, contains sound.

If you have the sense that the mind has wandered, or followed a particular sound into a memory or association, just notice where you went, and then bring your attention right back to receiving the sounds as the simple vibrations that they are.

Notice the interplay of the sounds in your environment. If you catch the mind labeling any of the sounds—like "door slamming," "bird singing," "neighbor's footstep above"—just notice that you've named the sound and then gently draw your awareness back. Let the vibrations exist as sound waves that are creating a general soundscape.

It's normal for the mind to want to attach stories or stimulate emotional responses as you passively receive different sound information. Take notice of that reaction. And then, without any judgment, just bring your focus back. You are only receiving sound—it enters the ears and then it fades away.

You may also notice the spaces between the sounds. And the unlikely "noise" sound within these quiet spaces. Allow your very sensitive microphone to pick up even the most subtle of vibrations in your soundscape right now. Different tones, volumes, lengths. Overlapping and one after another. Some melding together and some very distinct. Can you allow the sounds to simply come and go, without being concerned about their beginning or ending?

If you get a bit carried away in any one direction, or feel ungrounded, you can always come back to the sensation of the breath, breathing the body. Ground yourself for a moment and then return to the auditory input.

Observe the sound information entering your consciousness and then making its way out again. Practice experiencing sound as just pure vibration. With no thinking attached.

When you feel ready, begin to gently guide your attention back into the center of the chest. Place it on the rising and falling of the breath. Feel the weight of your body in the seat.

And then slowly begin to come back into the room, opening your eyes gently. And notice how you feel right now.

Part 2

Find a comfortable seated position, letting your spine lift up so it is very tall and spacious, and making the back of the neck as long as possible. With the legs and arms comfortable, and the hands resting softly on the lap, let the whole body relax gently into the seat. Close your eyes.

Place your attention right in the center of the chest now, and follow that rising and falling motion. Follow the natural pace and rhythm of the breath now, without trying to change it. Feel into any movement that it causes in the body—in the back, around the rib cage, the belly, or anywhere else you can sense it.

Now begin to expand your awareness, gradually making it a little wider, drawing it out a little more until the entire body falls within the scope of your focus.

Feel the effect of the breathing throughout the entire body now, as a whole—as if the air coming in and going out is breathing the entire body. Without trying to change it, just notice this constancy, the flow, the undulations. Inquire into their qualities.

Now gently begin to guide your attention away from the body and breath to the sounds coming in from the environment around you. Slowly focus your full attention on the soundscape—the various sounds and vibrations that are active in your environment right now.

You may notice the sounds in the room you're sitting in—the slight buzzing of electricity, an air conditioner or heater, the creaking of a floor or door. Or if there's quiet and stillness, perhaps you can hear the sound of your own breathing. You may observe sounds that are occurring outside the room, outside the building you're in—people talking, automobiles, birds, airplanes, wind, rain... Try not to reach for any sound. Your role is to be a sensitive receiver. Allow all sounds to simply exist in your awareness as vibration.

Curb any desire to explore why a certain sound is present, or create any story behind it. Simply receive all the different types of vibrations as they pop up in your awareness and as they drift away again.

Notice the details of each different vibration—the pitch, the distance from your ears, the volume, the duration of the sound. Take note of any other details you can recognize.

When multiple sounds are occurring at once, your focus may hone in on one sound and then shift to another. Watch how this process occurs. Your attention may also gather all the sounds that are present and witness them as one grand soundscape around you. Take a curious interest in how this may occur.

Notice the way in which you naturally pick up these vibrations.

And if you see the mind beginning to label any of the sounds, or attach a story or an emotion to them, see if you can simply notice that this has happened and then bring yourself back. Just refocusing on that very raw sensation—that very natural sense of vibration itself.

Now gently guide your attention back to the breath—the rising and falling movement. Allow all sound and vibration to release, and just follow your own natural breath. Feeling it again as it moves the body slightly. Feeling its pulse, its lifting and falling.

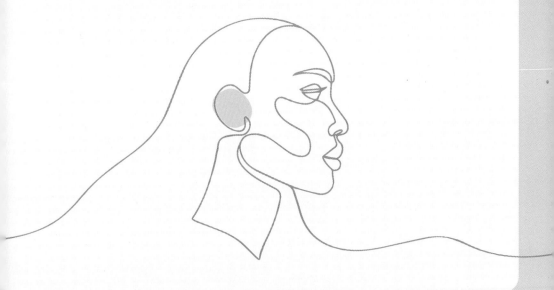

Prepare to come back into the physical space by sensing your body weight in the chair or on the cushion once again. Notice briefly the feeling of the air on the face and skin, and then allow your eyes to open slowly. Before moving on, just notice how you feel.

Part 3

Find a comfortable seated position where the spine can be tall with the head floating on top. Find a softness, but an alertness within your posture. Close your eyes.

Now turn your attention inward to your breath, directing it right into the center of the chest. Attending only to this natural rhythm now, with a one-pointed focus. Follow the feeling of the breath as it is right now.

For a few moments, steadily observe the breath in its natural state.

When you feel ready, begin to expand the awareness to view the body as a whole. See this breath starting to communicate now with the body as a whole. Just watching, just noticing.

Now direct your awareness from the body and breath to the sounds that are coming in from your environment—whatever sounds exist there right now. All of your

focus is now on receiving sound in the form of simple vibration. See what sounds you notice coming in and going back out. Do they feel any particular way? They may be coming from far off in the distance— like an airplane flying by, a siren, children playing in the park. Or they may be closer sounds—the humming of your computer, footsteps, water running in the next room. Notice any and all sounds... without reaching for them. Simply stay in your center and allow the reception of sound to take place.

If you catch yourself thinking or wondering about a particular sound, just notice where the mind has gone. Notice that the mind may have wanted to label a sensation and become involved with a story about the sensation. Just notice, do not judge. Once you've noticed, simply bring your attention back to this light, soft awareness.

Just witnessing, just observing sound coming in and going out. Without any associations. Just sound in its most basic, organic form—vibration.

What else do you notice? Engage your inner scientist. Does your brain tend to receive sound like an orchestra? Gathering and merging distinct sources of sound into one singular soundscape? Or is your attention more inclined to hone in on individual sounds as they make their way through, switching from one to another?

The moment you notice the mind getting involved with personalizing a sound, come right back to the more general sensation again. Just as if you were watching clouds float by in the sky, some moving fast, some moving slow. Some moving in groups, some individually. Dark clouds, light clouds, and clouds of all different shapes. It is all happening independently of you. You are just observing what is taking place.

And if you get taken away too far into thought, then come back to the body and breath for a moment—use the breath as your anchor. Then, as soon as you can, gently guide yourself back to the passive awareness of sound as ever-changing vibration.

And now start to bring your attention back, all of your attention—right into the center of the chest. Feel the breath moving there, up and down. In and out. Feel the body again in its seat. And begin to come back into the room by slowly opening your eyes. Take a moment here to notice exactly how you feel.

Change the scene

Try moving this practice into different environments if possible. For example, a more natural or secluded outdoor location will provide a very different experience than a busy public space. Practicing in your home or work environment will be very different to practicing in a new location that provides novel stimuli. Try to practice in a variety of places and notice any differences.

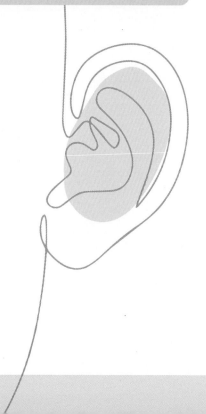

4

Mindful Awareness of Thoughts

Watching our own thoughts without actively thinking/engaging with them is one of the most challenging mindfulness practices for most people. We are very inclined to get carried away with our own stories, reasoning, emotional triggers, and self-judgment. Self-compassion and kindness is encouraged in every meditation practice, but is especially important when you are becoming familiar with, and accepting, the thoughts that are continually active in the psyche.

Three-part meditation

Takes 5–20 minutes

Level Beginner to Intermediate

Preparation Find any comfortable seated position on a chair or a cushion on the floor.

Part 1

Settle into a comfortable seated position with the spine straight. Your body should feel relaxed, yet alert. Let any stress or fatigue roll away, and then close your eyes.

Just begin by taking several slow, deep breaths, inhaling all the way down to the belly and exhaling back up and out. On each exhale, let the body sink into its comfortable seat or position a little more.

Now let the breath return to its natural rhythm. Without trying to change the breath, just see it fall right back into its natural pace. A feeling of gentle alertness enters the body on each inhale, and a grounding, softening of the body on each exhale. Let any remaining tension flow out until you sense that the body and the breath are in their natural state of being.

Create an image in your mind now to guide your focus inward. You can imagine this is happening at the back of the forehead. Pretend you have a movie screen or a blank canvas there, and mentally draw the image. This could be something simple—like a flower, a mountain top, or the face of someone you care for. Choose one thing, and whatever it is, try to see it there in your mind's eye in as much detail as you can.

Don't be discouraged if this doesn't come easily at first, just keep gently re-making the image. When the picture dissipates, just continue to watch with your attention softly in this same location. Then, before the mind can wander, try to recreate the picture once more. The goal is to keep your full focus on the arena of the mind, but, again, try not to get involved with what appears.

Notice that just as every breath will come and go, and information from the five senses will come and go, so will mental images and thoughts. Coming and going of their own accord. You don't need to try to change them, understand them, latch onto them, or push them away. Just practice observing this mental movie screen—by simply watching.

The images being projected here may seem crucial or perhaps emotionally-charged. They may also be random and feel disconnected from you. Sometimes there may be no mental impressions appearing at all for some time. All of these experiences are normal.

Let whatever may be there just be there. Without needing to analyze, or getting drawn into any particular thought or feeling, just allow yourself to notice the images as they come and go. As if you were watching clouds floating by in the sky. Watching from a bit of a distance, remaining unconcerned.

Depending on your current conditions, which vary from day-to-day, the mind may behave differently. It may look very active and alive, or it may seem very still. Try to regard both as the same. Without critique. Try your best to remain neutral, just observing what takes place when you rest your awareness in the mental space where thoughts appear and disappear.

If you notice the mind following or getting heavily involved with any particular thought, just take a mental step back. Pause and observe every image as impermanent—just like a cloud in the sky or a ripple on the water. Some stay a little longer, and some move by quite quickly. All passing through eventually within your field of awareness.

As the breath naturally rises and falls, so will the thoughts in the mind. Rising and falling endlessly in our waking hours. Appearing and disappearing. Take the

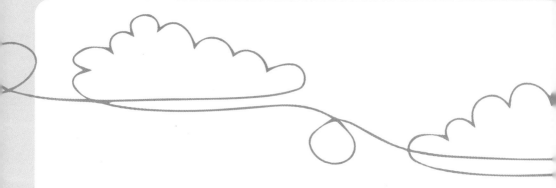

perspective of viewing all of the activity together—as if you were gazing out at waves coming into shore and then flowing back out to sea.

Just watching, with no need to get involved. And really noticing with a sense of curiosity the types of thoughts that stop by, how long they stay for, and also the sensation of stillness and space between each one.

When you inevitably feel that you're being taken away by a particular stream of thinking, then, on your next inhale, allow the breath energy to return you to your center. The center seat in the theater of the mind. Just watching any action or non-action.

If you notice any physical sensations drawing your attention away, do your best to let them go on the next exhale. Soften the body back into stillness, then return your awareness back to watching the mind.

There is no right or wrong. Just as we watched the body, noticing its qualities; and studied the breath, noticing its

sensations and rhythms; and allowed sounds to come and go, in the same way we're just gazing into this play of mental activity that is not "us" but is always taking place for us.

Now very slowly start to shift your attention back to your breath, feeling it rising and falling again, sensing it moving the body gently.

Feel the body and its weight, its points of contact with the seat. Begin to open your eyes slowly. And take a moment just to notice how you feel right now.

Part 2

Find a comfortable position for the body where the spine can be erect and the chest gently lifted. As much as possible, encourage the body to be alert, yet soft and relaxed. Allow your eyes to close.

Start to take a few nice deep breaths, breathing all the way down into the belly and then all the way back up and out. Release any residual tension and relax

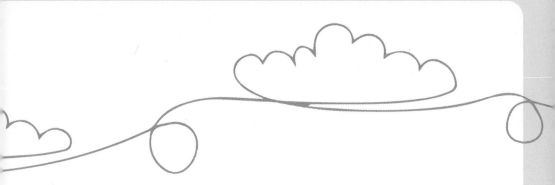

more on each exhale. Then let the breath return to its normal pace.

Start to shift your attention up now to the mental space—the area where all images and thoughts arise. You may want to start by creating an image in your mind to bring your focus directly to this area. Imagine now seeing a simple, familiar image behind the forehead, somewhere inside the skull. Let your attention gather and settle in this space.

Now whatever image you chose, see it there in precise detail, as if you're viewing a photograph in your mind. Now watch it for as long as it wants to stay. And when the image begins to fade away, allow it to dissipate—don't struggle with it, don't try to hang on to it. Let it go and leave your attention right there, in that space.

Without any sense of reaching or searching, now allow any thoughts, memories, fantasies, or daydreams to pass by, in their own time. All mental activity just flowing in and out at its own natural rhythm, by itself. Become the observer. You can imagine you're seated a little ways

back from this movie screen of your mind. In this mental space, this arena where all thoughts and images interplay—there is no right or wrong.

You are not doing the projecting. You are simply watching the show. Noticing what comes, with the intention not to get involved. Without the desire to like or dislike any particular thought, pattern, or feeling that reveals itself.

Remain in a neutral space, comfortably seated in the mental theater and viewing the appearances of the mind, of the subconscious, with a childlike curiosity.

You may notice your thoughts come in different guises—as daydreams, anticipations about the future, memories of things that happened this morning or last week. However they come, simply do your best to let them just be exactly as they are.

It's natural to notice yourself getting strongly drawn away by certain thoughts or feelings, but as soon as you notice this is happening, try to recenter yourself in that neutral space. In that settled, gentle awareness. Likewise, if the body calls your attention away with the five senses, just notice where your attention has gone and then gently release those physical sensations on your next out-breath. Return again to that comfortable seat in the space of the mind—just watching the show.

There is no need to interpret or figure anything out. Make peace with your true nature, the stillness that resides inside. Allow everything else to just come and go as it pleases.

When you're ready, allow all of the mental activity to subside by simply removing your attention. Bringing the attention back down into the body now, feeling the breath fully as it moves in and out.

Refocusing now on bodily sensations— the weight of your body in the seat, the feeling of the air on your skin and face. As your eyes begin to open, come back into the room gracefully. And just take a moment to notice how you feel.

Part 3

Find a comfortable position where the spine can be as long and straight as possible and the limbs relaxed. The body should feel soft, yet alert and aware. Begin by closing your eyes and bringing your attention to the breath.

Start with a few long, deep breaths, filling up completely with each inhale and releasing any remaining tension on your exhales.

Feel the body softening into its position even more as you allow your breath to return to its natural pace. Let your body decide whether the breath is fast or slow, regular or irregular now, and leave it be.

Start to move your awareness, all of your attention, to the mental space— that mental arena of your thoughts. Imagine this space as a wide-open sky. Clear and pristine. And you're sitting back comfortably, just viewing anything that takes place. Without any sort of judgment, without any need to figure anything out— let the mind be exactly as it is right now.

Your mind might be very active or impatient, and the thoughts may seem to be very concerning. Or your mind may be very still, and slow, and spacious. Try to release any sense of preference you feel you should have for one or the other. Just study the mind without scrutinizing. Watch with a soft curiosity. What is the quality of the mental activity? At what speed are thoughts coming and going? What types of thoughts stay around for longer, or which ones tend to repeat? Perhaps noticing where the thoughts seem to be coming from—from where do they arise? Are they coming from a space that seems separate from yourself? Where do they go when they disappear?

Continue to observe, all the while remaining detached. Stay in the neutral space of your calm awareness. The only task right now is simply to notice—notice the thoughts and the images, the stories, the concerns, the daydreams. Watch it all come and go, floating in and out of the open awareness that you've created.

See if the simple act of turning awareness upon a thought affects it—how does acknowledging it without trying to engage change its qualities? Cultivate an attitude of not wanting any particular experience. Instead, stay present with whatever arises.

When you do get taken away along a certain pathway, toward a certain thought process, just notice that your attention has wandered again and bring everything back a little further. Contract your awareness back into that calm space. Take a broader view of the content of the mind as it exists right now.

All mental images come and go naturally, constantly changing and adapting. And right now, you can just be the observer. Unconcerned.

Begin to let all thoughts subside as you move your fullest attention back to the breath. Feel the sensation of the air enter and exit the body again—the chest rising and falling. Notice the weight of your body, the points of contact with the seat. The sensations of the skin, the feeling of the face.

And start to open your eyes, bringing yourself back into the room. Take a moment here to notice any current feelings or sensations.

Thought patterns

Most humans have thousands of thoughts per day—many of these stem from subconscious, learned patterns. Many of them repeat over and over and over... and over.

We can learn to observe what sorts of thought patterns are prevalent in our own mind, practice accepting them, and, finally, work to incrementally change or replace the ones that aren't benefiting us anymore.

5

Mindful Eating

This exercise can help you get more in touch with the deeper, more meaningful aspects of nourishing yourself with food. It may also reveal a lot of useful information about your eating habits and preferences. Our attention is focused on the sensations that arise from the food and the body's reaction to seeing, smelling, chewing, and eating.

One-part meditation

Takes 5–10 minutes

Level Beginner

Preparation In this practice we use a piece of fruit (such as a segment of orange, a slice of apple, or a strawberry) as an anchor and the object of attention and exploration. Whatever you choose will be your "seed," or focus, for the meditation. Prepare something small and take a comfortable seat—as you would normally to eat a meal—on a chair at a table or on a cushion on the floor. Set the piece of fruit in front of you where you can see it.

Straighten your spine, relax your belly, and take three slow, deep breaths. Imagine completely releasing any tension from the body and mind with every exhale.

Now, gently gazing at the piece of fruit in front of you, begin to consider where it came from and how it made its way to your table. Where was it grown? In which country? Did it grow naturally outside or was it grown in a greenhouse?

Think about the people who may have grown your fruit—watering it and caring for it. Imagine the people who picked the fruit and who packaged it. Consider who transported this fruit from where it was grown and packaged to your location, and what it must have taken to get it there. And also consider the people who unpacked it at the store and placed it on the shelves... and those who sold it to you.

Imagine this whole process, the entire life cycle of the fruit before it even reached your hands and all the people who worked to provide you with this nourishment. Extend a sense of gratitude to all of them. As you proceed, notice if this feeling of being grateful for your food affects your experience of eating, and how.

Now pick up the piece of fruit and turn it over, examining it closely and looking at it as if you've never seen such a thing before. Gaze at it with new eyes. What colors do you notice? Are the colors consistent on each side?

What kinds of textures do you see and feel? Notice the weight of the fruit, the shape of the fruit—is this regular or irregular? Is the fruit a certain temperature?

Now bring the piece of fruit closer to your mouth, stopping just under your nose, and notice if it has a smell. If so, is the smell subtle or strong? And does this particular smell influence your thoughts or feelings (does it bring back any specific memories)?

Take a bite from the piece of fruit and place it on your tongue. But don't chew yet. Just let the fruit sit there for a moment and notice how the tongue and mouth respond to it. Notice if you have an urge to chew and then swallow quickly.

Now very slowly begin to chew the bite of fruit. Be aware of the texture and how it changes. Aware of all the different flavors and where on the tongue you are registering these flavors—can you make out sweet, sour, bitter?

Now swallow and, with your engaged attention, follow the food down as far as you can—down the throat and into the stomach. Notice what this feels like. Try to notice all of the sensations without being led away into memories or daydreams. Remain present to how the sensations shift as you chew and swallow.

Take a second bite from the piece of fruit and continue this present-awareness— from bringing the fruit under your nose to placing it in your mouth to swallowing it.

Continue eating slowly and notice if your experience of sensations changes from bite to bite, or if your desire to eat more quickly or more slowly shifts.

When you have finished, take a moment to close your eyes and just notice any flavors or sensations that still remain in the mouth or belly.

6

Mindfulness of Support from the Ground

Practicing mindfulness in a still, standing position gives us a different sensory experience to learn than that from a seated or moving meditation. Here we practice awareness of the body sensations in relation to support from the ground below us.

One-part meditation

Takes 5–10 minutes

Level Beginner

Preparation Practice this exercise somewhere quiet. Whether indoors, or out in nature or a quiet section of the park, try to find a location where you won't be disturbed for at least five minutes.

Find a natural standing position. Try not to think about this too much, as there is no right or wrong here. Close your eyes and take a moment to just feel your body as it stands still, finding its own natural resting point.

Now make any minor adjustments to ensure you are as comfortable as possible, so you can continue the exercise from a place of pure observation and curiosity, without moving around.

Feel the feet grounded down onto the floor or ground, and notice the sturdiness of the legs and how the rest of the body balances right on top.

Notice the position of the head, shoulders, hips, and knees... all the way down to the feet.

Observe how the soles of the feet feel right now. Where are the strongest points of contact with the floor or ground? Is your body weight falling equally across the feet or is it leaning more on the right or the left foot?

Investigate whether the weight falls more to the outside or inside of the feet, more toward the heels or the toes, or if it feels evenly distributed between the right and left sides. What other sensations can you pinpoint?

See how the ankles and legs feel in this moment. Check in with the hips and pelvis. Notice any information from the body, without moving, shifting, or changing position. Continue scanning up the body with your focused attention, without any sense of judgment for what you may find, until you eventually come to the top of the head.

For a moment, expand your attention so that it zooms out and can encompass your entire body, as a whole. What does your entire body, as a singular, cooperative unit, feel like at this moment?

Now take a moment to extend your awareness back into the room or immediate surrounding area and slowly begin to engage with all of your senses.

Notice the objects surrounding you, and any colors, sounds, or smells within your sphere. Take in the general tone of the environment. Notice how you feel.

Focus on the body

This exercise is another version of a body scan, or bringing acute mindfulness to the body's sensations. To expand on this experience, try bringing your attention to the breath, or the sounds in your environment, or your train of thought instead.

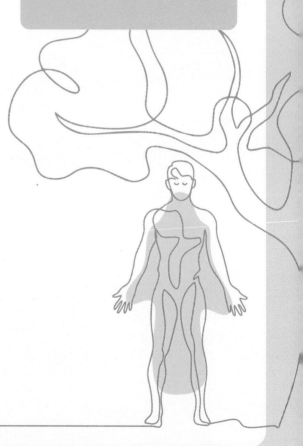

7

Mindfulness of Walking

Like mindfulness in standing, but more dynamic, this exercise allows you to witness a larger array of sensations and adjustments in the body and its rhythms as you naturally shift your weight and guide your body through space.

One-part meditation

Takes 5–10 minutes

Level Beginner

Preparation Find an indoor or outdoor space large enough to walk in large circles, be this the perimeter of a room or around a tree in the park. If it feels comfortable, take your shoes off to ground and connect even more.

Start to walk at a very comfortable pace, but one that's a little slower than you would usually use in your need to "get somewhere." Notice how the feet move— one foot touching down at the heel and rolling toward the toes, just as the other lifts up and comes forward to touch down at the heel and again rolls toward the toes.

Try to imagine it is your first time walking, that you've never walked before. Infuse your attention with a child-like curiosity. Simply notice how this action feels...

Notice where the weight is in your left foot when the right lifts up... and where the weight is in your right foot when the left lifts up...

Without trying to change anything, and without critiquing or judging, just rest your awareness on the natural, synchronous movements as you walk.

Now notice the feeling of the legs moving along with the feet. What sensations exist there? And the movement of the hips, back and forth, or side to side. Notice how the body may move and shift in response to each step to maintain balance. Observe the torso... see the arms swinging gently, automatically. Witness the shoulders, the neck and head.

Continue to walk, slowly and mindfully, with the intention of simply being present and experiencing the wonder of walking that we so often take for granted. Rest your attention down at your feet as they lift, move forward, and touch down to the floor or ground again, while remaining alert to any emotions, thoughts, or memories that may come up or flow by your conscious awareness. Watch them lightly as well, without getting involved.

After 5–10 minutes, or once the process feels complete for you, take a comfortable seat and notice how you feel for a moment or two.

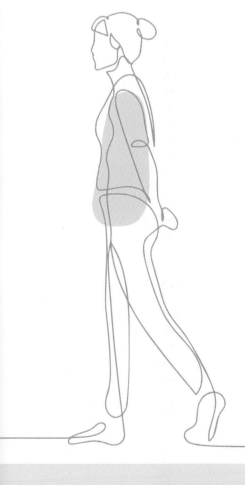

On the move

This exercise can be translated into an everyday-life mindful moment. Anytime you're walking and decide to "check in," take a moment to slow down, focus your attention on the sensations of walking, and watch any particular thoughts or emotions that may come up, but without engaging with them. Every time you walk is an opportunity to return to mindfulness and to engage with the present moment rather than allowing repetitive thoughts or worries to lead you on your path.

8

Mindfulness of Compassion

Compassion meditation helps us to get back in touch with our sense of empathy and the experience of outflowing positive thoughts and wishes to oneself and others. Through practice it can help us find ways to connect when we feel isolated, to let go of judgment, and to find forgiveness— which is one of the most healing gifts that we can give to ourselves.

Two-part meditation

Takes 5–20 minutes

Level Beginner to Advanced

Preparation Either seated or lying on your back, find a comfortable position where your spine can be straight. If you're sitting in a chair, let your feet be grounded, with arms resting comfortably and palms on the lap. If you're seated on the floor, you can cross your legs and bring your hands to any mudra, or position, you wish to use (a mudra is a position or shape made with the hands and fingers that's meant to focus the energy in particular ways). If you're lying on a bed, keep the legs straight with the arms away from the body and the palms up, or rest the hands on the heart center.

Part 1

Once you're comfortable, allow any extra stress or fatigue to just roll off and away from the shoulders. Start to tune into your breath. Become familiar with how the breath feels and how it's moving right now. With no concern for changing it, no need to alter it in any way—just keeping watch.

Now very slowly begin to extend your breaths so that your inhales and exhales are an equal, steady length. Breathing through the nose, in and out—slow and calm—but natural. Breathing in and out for about the same length of time now.

Now let the breath be. Bring your focus to your heart center, and feel the rising and falling motion there, at the very center of the chest. Watch the movement already taking place, on its own.

Start to imagine an energy gathering in and around the heart center. See it as a colorful radiance gathering there—use any color that pops into your head or perhaps a ball of bright white light, or any other way that helps you. Allow this energy to continue gathering there... getting stronger and more dense with each in-breath.

Bring someone to mind that you know well and would like to see receive a positive turn of events or good fortune. Try to see them in your mind's eye with as much detail as possible—like viewing a photograph. See them looking back at you and smiling, making eye contact. Focus here until you have a strong image of this person (and perhaps an emotional response to the image in your body—like a softening of your shoulders or a slight organic smile).

Now transfer this energy to them. Just imagining that it is happening is enough. See that energy built up around your heart now traveling in real-time to this person, and watch them gratefully absorb and accept it with joy. Allow yourself to enjoy the giving, and get the strong sense that this person will use this extra energy for their highest good.

When this process feels complete for you, simply turn your attention back to the rising and falling of the breath. Start to notice the weight of your body in the chair, or on the floor or bed. Sense the air on the skin and face, preparing to come back into the room. When you're ready, gently open your eyes. Take a moment to notice how you feel.

Part 2

Find a comfortable position, close your eyes softly, and begin to let yourself unfold and release any remaining tension.

We'll begin by bringing to mind one aspect, one part of yourself that you love. Decide on just one thing for this exercise (you can add more next time). It should be something about yourself that you honor, that you are proud of. It could be a good deed that you did, a decision that you are proud of, or just any quality that you really like about yourself. Don't worry if there is resistance the first few times you do this exercise—the more you practice, the easier it will become. It will become more and more natural to focus on your self-value. If nothing comes to mind right away, don't worry—just rest in the fact that you have the desire to be happy.

Just focus on the positive feeling or sensation—even if it is mild right now—and see it breathing, beating, expanding there at the center of the chest. Allow your breath to just flow in and out now in this relaxed state. Once your attention is steady and focused on or near the heart center, repeat these phrases mentally, keeping as open a mind as possible:

I am Well.
I am Happy.
I am Peaceful.
I am Loved.

Repeat the phrases twice more to yourself, trying to feel the vibration of the words and the intentions behind them building and warming near your heart.

Next, bring to mind someone you have a positive association with or share positive feelings with—this could be a friend, family member, or teacher. Picture them clearly, either by imagining them right in front of you or visualizing them in your mind's eye. Try to see all the details of their face.

Now send out the same messages directly to that person—mentally:

May You be Well.
May You be Happy.
May You be Peaceful.
May You be Loved.

Imagine the pure kindness of this intention flowing swiftly toward them... Repeat the messages twice more.

Imagine you can see the energy reaching out from you across space, to reach this person, and watch as it is accepted and absorbed. Again, repeat twice more.

Now bring to mind someone who you have no particular feeling for or against—someone neutral. This could be a cashier, someone you see occasionally on your walk to work, etc. Someone with no positive or negative emotional connection—as neutral as possible. Bring them to mind with as much detail as possible, and recite mentally:

May You be Well.
May You be Happy.
May You be Peaceful.
May You be Loved.

Watch them receiving all of the benefits, all of the goodness of this message, this energy. Repeat the messages twice more.

Lastly, imagine someone who you're currently having a difficult time with. Think of a more challenging relationship or someone who you've had a disagreement with. When you think of this person you may feel a palpable sense of conflict or uneasiness. That's okay. Try to bring them to mind anyway, in the most gentle way possible, and, knowing that your personal well of compassion is infinitely deep, send them this message now:

May You be Well.
May You be Happy.
May You be Peaceful.
May You be Loved.

Don't worry if this feels challenging at first. Just trust that you're sending the best energy you can, that the person is able to receive it, and that they are doing so with grace.

Realize the sensations occurring in your own body and spirit—the truly unlimited energy that is radiating from your heart.

And without any expectation, direct the same message toward this person:

> *May You be Well.*
> *May You be Happy.*
> *May You be Peaceful.*
> *May You be Loved.*

No matter what the circumstance is, just keep sending the message unconditionally. Focusing on the expansiveness of your own heart and how wide your sphere of compassion can grow. Repeat the messages twice more.

Now, just for a moment, see this energy outflowing to all three of these people, while at the same time multiplying within your own being. Notice the expansive quality of this present moment. When you open your eyes, try to focus on this sensation and take it with you out into the world, for the rest of the day. Practice freely extending it to others and dually embracing it for yourself.

The source of wellbeing
All beings desire these traits: to be healthy, to be happy, to live in peace, and to experience love and equanimity. Know that your own personal source of wellbeing is full—right at the center of the heart. The more that you extend love and compassion to others, the more love and compassion you'll be able to receive in your own life.

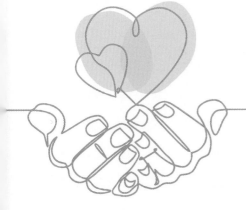

9

Mindful Listening & Communication

Listening to someone speak may seem like a natural, passive mode of communication, but when we begin to pay attention, we notice that we are often hearing what someone is saying on one level, while we run our own internal narrative on another. In addition to our own mental distractions and swirling thoughts, our emotions tend to get involved and can cause internal reactions to the speaker's words that may have nothing to do with what they're trying to express. We have the urge to respond right away, to make our point or express our opinion. Or to soothe or assist. Or perhaps just to guess the endpoint and bring the conversation to an end. Because of the nature of the mind and its conditioning to interrupt or interject, we often never receive the complete communication that the other was trying to express. Our attention is normally too divided.

Mindful listening allows us the space to give the other's words, as well as the energy and expression behind their words, our full and unwavering attention. Rather than staying in a reactive mode, we actively stay in a receptive mode so that we can truly hear the other person.

Two-part meditation

Takes 5–20 minutes

Level Beginner to Intermediate

Preparation Sit comfortably back-to-back on chairs or cushions on the floor. You'll need a timer, plus a pen and notebook or some scrap paper for each person to journal in.

Part 1

For this practice you don't need anything special except a nonjudgmental attitude and the willingness to cultivate patience and self-reflection while listening to others in normal daily conversations. Listening can be a challenge, especially in today's fast-moving, attention-split world.

To practice listening more mindfully, conduct some brief check-ins during normal conversations and notice what you're thinking about. Here are some questions to reflect upon during and after a conversation:

- Are you thinking about what the speaker is saying throughout the whole conversation?
- Has the mind wandered off into another story about the things they're saying?
- Has the mind activated a story that is hardly related but which you were reminded of?
- How quickly do you recognize this when it happens?
- Are there periods when you're so distracted by someone else's conversation or a noise or event in your environment that you completely lose track of the speaker's words and have to ask them to repeat themselves or clarify?
- Are there points in the conversation where you stop actually hearing the person speak?
- What does your internal dialogue look like and how does it behave once you notice it over the speaker's words?
- Do you feel the need to respond, react, defend, inform, or change the topic? Why?

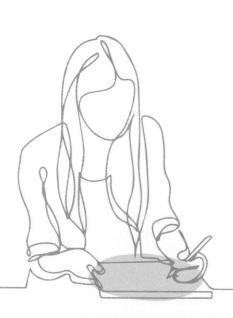

Part 2

Reflective Listening

This exercise is practiced with a partner. Sitting comfortably back-to-back, the partners take turns speaking about anything they like for exactly two minutes. During the two minutes the speaker can talk about the past, the present, or the future. They can have periods of silence if that feels right. There's no right or wrong subject matter here. The focus is to just talk about whatever presents itself in the speaker's mind, and to let things flow naturally without any sense of forcing words or stories to come. The partner that is listening says nothing and remains perfectly quiet, without acknowledging or replying to what their partner is saying. They are just there, mindfully receiving the storyline, the emotional undertones, and anything else they can sense about the communication for the duration of the two minutes. If not responding at all to the storyteller proves too difficult, you can also agree on one phrase to acknowledge that the listener understands what the speaker is saying (such as "I understand" or "uh-huh").

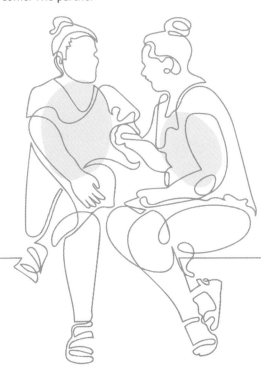

Make sure to use a timer. When the two minutes is up, the partner who was listening begins to speak. Their goal is simply to state what they heard their partner saying, using the phrase "I heard you say that..." They are simply reflecting back what they perceived. For example, "I heard you say that your work environment is frustrating and the stress is spilling over into your home life..."; "I heard you say that your relationship feels secure..." or whatever it is that they heard their partner communicating.

Now each partner can take five minutes and free-journal about their experience and insights. Set the timer again and just write anything that comes to mind, anything that may have stood out for you about your perceptions or your communication style.

Now, switch partners. Again sitting back-to-back, now the listener is the speaker and the speaker listens without the need to interrupt. Set the timer for two minutes and allow the speaker the entire time period to express anything that's on their mind. When the time is up, the listener will reflect back what they heard the speaker say, and then each person should take another five minutes to free-write about what they experienced.

This is a powerful exercise because it makes us mindful of how we listen to others—are we truly listening, or just planning a response, following a memory, or planning for later in the day?

It also makes us aware of how and to what extent we are heard by others—are we expressing ourselves and our intentions clearly? Are we getting our point across without struggle?

Mindfulness in the everyday

As you are beginning to see, mindfulness grows through instilling awareness into everyday activities. Making a series of small shifts can create a large impact on how you relate to the world and others in it.

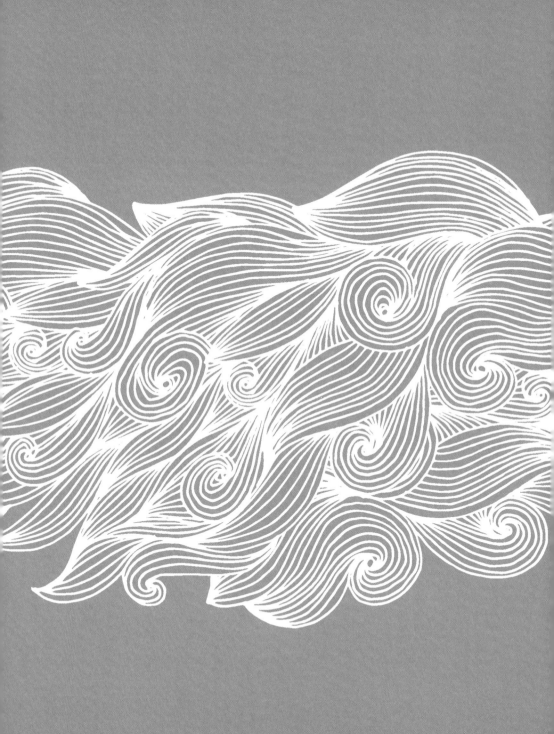

CHAPTER 2
CALM

Why are calming, stress-reducing meditations
important and how do they work? While it
may be true that many types of meditation
can have the positive side effect of stress
relief, there are specific meditation techniques
that can help induce a calm, serene state
very quickly and deeply.

Finding Calm

The practices in this chapter have the power to lower the heart rate and reduce blood pressure, to tame inflammation throughout the body, and even to boost our immune systems.

Methods of controlling or slowing down the breath as well as visualization exercises can swiftly activate the parasympathetic nervous system, also called the Rest and Digest mode of our autonomic nervous system (the part of the nervous system that directs and controls subconscious body activity such as digestion, hormone release, and much more).

When our system is calm we can more easily find moments of mental and emotional rest as well, and more of our sleep becomes truly restorative. Chronic stress keeps the nervous system "hijacked" and in Fight or Flight mode, but when we practice deep relaxation we give the body a chance to find homeostasis and balance itself out, on both a micro and macro level. Turbulent emotions can be eased, a racing mind can be stilled, daily energy levels can be restored, and much more.

Many of these techniques have been used for decades in the sciences of psychology, Western medicine, and alternative healing, and also in professional training for sports, dance, and the arts. What can be imagined and practiced can be strengthened. By practicing getting into and remaining comfortable in relaxed states, one can actually rewire the brain so that it feels more relaxed and serene, more of the time. Over time, neural networks are redesigned and new connections are built that can help remove stress from all of our bodily systems as well as from our relationships with ourselves and others.

Many of these techniques have been used for decades in the sciences of psychology, Western medicine, and alternative healing, and also in professional training for sports, dance, and the arts.

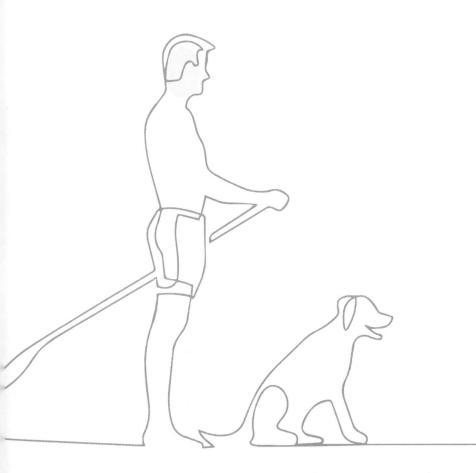

10

Calming Breath

This breath directs your attention inside to the physical anchor of the breath. By counting the breath we can make the inhales and exhales truly equal—balancing the mind and body quite quickly, to bring about a profound sense of calm. The breath often slows down of its own accord, and we can notice and feel the spaces between the breaths. We can then explore that serene space by lengthening its pause as well.

Three-part meditation

Takes 5–15 minutes

Level Beginner

Preparation Find any comfortable seated position on a chair or a cushion on the floor, where the spine and chest are lifted and the belly is soft.

Part 1

Once you've found a comfortable seat, and the body is relaxed yet alert, allow your eyes to close softly and bring your attention inward to the breath.

Gradually begin to slow the breath down, creating inhales and exhales that are an equal length.

Allow the air to move down into the lowest part of the belly if this feels comfortable, and fill every corner of the torso, the rib cage, the chest. Fill up fully, but softly, so there's no sense of strain.

Begin now to count your in- and out-breaths mentally, adjusting the pace of the counting so it's comfortable and natural, yet just a tad slower than your normal breath might be. We'll start with 4 counts in and 4 counts back out of an equal and steady length. To begin, exhale completely.

Now inhale to a count of 4:

1-2-3-4

Exhale now for the same number of counts:

1-2-3-4

Continue in this way:

Inhaling 1-2-3-4
and
Exhaling 1-2-3-4

If you like, close your eyes to bring more focus to the breath sensations.

Continue on, gently breathing in for 4 counts and out for 4 counts.

Consciously slowing the breath down stimulates the part of our nervous system that is responsible for Rest and Digest mode—the parasympathetic nervous system. This is the state we're in when we're deeply relaxed. When we're asleep. When there's no fear. No stress. No worry or concern. Blood pressure is reduced, stress hormones become inactive, and the body begins to prepare itself for deep healing and rest. When we obtain this deep relaxation state, the body is prepared to rejuvenate on a cellular level. With

regular practice, the benefits can extend all the way out to the mental, emotional, and spiritual aspects of our being.

Continue these long, even breaths, counting to 4, with the awareness that you are encouraging the body to let go and renew. If any thoughts come into the mind during the breathing, just acknowledge them and allow them to release, like clouds floating away into the distant sky. This is a completely normal activity of the mind. Without concern or judgment, just keep returning your attention to the breath, counting slowly and evenly.

The next time you exhale completely, let your breath return to its normal, natural pace.

Take notice of how the body is feeling right now. How did the calming breathing affect your system, your physical structure, your mentality and mood?

And, when you're ready, slowly open your eyes. Take a moment to get familiar with and appreciate this sense of calm. With gratitude, acknowledge the time you've taken for yourself.

The more regularly you practice this exercise, the more easily you'll be able to return to this serene state of being—both during meditation and in everyday life.

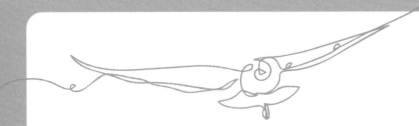

Part 2

Once you've found a comfortable seat, gently close your eyes. Allow the breath to become long and slow. Make the inhales and exhales an even length.

Think about softening your shoulders down away from your ears, softening your palms, your hips, and any other place that you may be feeling tension in the body right now.

Notice your breath as it begins to slow, moving all the way down into your belly. With every exhale, the muscles get softer and softer.

In a moment, we'll begin to inhale the breath to a count of 4 and exhale the breath to a count of 4.

Let's begin. Exhale all the air out.

Inhale now 1-2-3-4
and
Exhale 1-2-3-4

Inhale 1-2-3-4
and
Exhale 1-2-3-4

Continue on your own now, inhaling for 4 and exhaling for 4, slowly and smoothly.

Start to notice the slight pause at the top of each inhale—that little space before the exhale begins again. Bring your attention to that moment between the in- and out-breath. Notice the quality of that space, the stillness there. Likewise, at the bottom of each exhale, notice that moment before the next inhale takes place. Notice the quality of this pause— the silence, the comfort, the neutrality.

Begin now to gently extend those spaces between each breath for one extra count. Just lightly suspending the pause, without gripping or creating tension. Feel the lengthening of the natural space between the ins and outs.

Inhaling for 4, suspending for 1, exhaling for 4, suspending for 1, and so on.

Continue in this manner if the breath still feels comfortable. And, with a childlike curiosity, continue to look into the sense of stillness that already exists there between every single breath.

The next time you exhale, allow your breath to return to its normal rhythm. Just a nice, natural pace. Notice any sensations or feelings in the body. Notice any sense of calm or peacefulness that may have taken root.

When you're ready, slowly open your eyes. Take a moment to get familiar with and appreciate this sense of calm.

With gratitude, acknowledge the time you've taken for yourself and know that the more you practice this exercise, the more quickly and easily you'll be able to return to this serene state of being.

Part 3

Find a comfortable position where the spine can be as straight as possible, and where the body can relax and soften.

Draw your attention toward your breath, and the constant movement of air through the physical body. Notice the rise and fall, the inward and outward motion.

Without changing anything, just notice any qualities of the breath that stand out to you right now. Does the breath feel full, shallow? Fast or slow? Cool or warm? Where is the breath traveling within

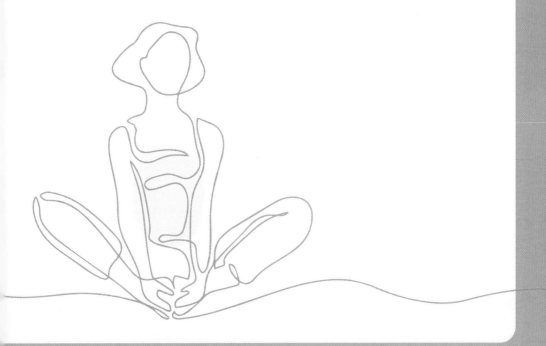

your body? Is it freely filling the whole of your lungs and rib cage? Can you feel the breath reach down to the belly? To the pelvis or hips? Does it flow into the side-body? Or into the back-body, toward the shoulder blades? Just notice how the breath is behaving, right now, at this point in time.

In a moment, we'll begin counting the breath with a pattern of 8-4-8. The inhale will be for a count of 8, and then we'll gently hold, suspending the breath at the top of the inhale for 4 counts, before exhaling again to a count of 8. (If you like, you can add a slight pause, or one count, at the bottom of each exhale as in the previous exercise, but this isn't necessary. Just use your own discretion.)

Let's begin together. Exhale completely.

Inhale through the nose
1-2-3-4-5-6-7-8
Hold softly
1-2-3-4
Exhale through the nose
1-2-3-4-5-6-7-8

Inhale
1-2-3-4-5-6-7-8
Hold softly
1-2-3-4
Exhaling
1-2-3-4-5-6-7-8

Continue this pattern on your own, continuing to count 8-4-8. If at any point you lose track of the counting, just start over at the next inhale. Make the breath slow and steady. Nothing forced. Just a comfortable breath and a soft, gentle hold. No gripping in the throat, no strain or pressure building up. Just gently extend the natural pause for 4 counts between the inhales and exhales.

For the next few minutes continue breathing in the pattern 8-4-8.

If you notice any tension or pain present itself in the physical body, just acknowledge it and allow it to release, and then return your attention right back to the prescribed breathing pattern.

The next time you exhale, let the breath come back to normal. Release the counting. Let everything return to its natural state. With your attention still inward, watch the state of the breath as it relates to the state of the body and the state of the mind.

Notice how you feel. What are the qualities of the breath in this moment? Has anything shifted in your experience? There is no right or wrong, but practice inquiring about even subtle changes.

When you're ready, allow your eyes to softly float open. Take a moment to enjoy this feeling—with gratitude, acknowledge the time you've taken for yourself.

Know that the more you practice this exercise, the more quickly and easily you'll be able to return to this peaceful place, and the more deeply the internal healing will take place.

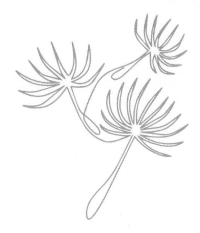

Tip

If holding the breath for 4 counts feels in any way uncomfortable or overly challenging, then reduce the count to 2. Also adjust the speed of the counts as needed. It's very important that there is no sense of strain or tension created from the exercise, as this counteracts any positive benefits for the nervous system. Every individual may require a slightly different breath length, and one length may feel good one day and bad the next. Be mindful about how you're feeling as you begin the exercise, and adjust as needed to find a count that you can maintain comfortably.

11

Stress Reduction SSS-Breath

One way to relax quickly is to make the exhale a little longer than the inhale. This helps to stimulate the vagus nerve, which brings the parasympathetic nervous system into play almost immediately. This exercise asks you to extend your exhale quite a bit, but in a very gentle and controlled manner. The exhale consists of a small but steady stream of air and the white-noise sound that's produced can serve as a tool to relax you even more deeply.

One-part meditation

Takes 5 minutes

Level Beginner

Preparation Stand or find any comfortable seated position on a chair or a cushion on the floor, ensuring the spine and chest are lifted, the shoulders back, and the belly soft. You can also lie on your back.

You can do this exercise standing up, seated, or lying down. Whatever your position, try to keep your back upright and chest slightly lifted so that the rib cage is spacious and the lungs can expand freely.

Begin with three deep, full inhales and exhales through the nose to ground and connect to your breath. Now fill up the lungs completely with fresh air.

Through the mouth, with the teeth close together and the tongue raised up toward the roof of the mouth, exhale very slowly and steadily, making a slight hissing or whispering sound as the air passes through. The exhale is controlled and smooth, and also audible.

It can help to think of a balloon in the abdomen—full of air, but with a pinprick in the side so that the air can escape quite passively, smoothly, and gradually.

As you practice this breath, the muscles used in breathing—especially the diaphragm—will become strong and conditioned. This will make the exhale consistent and controlled, creating an exhale that is much longer than the inhale, stimulating an immediate response from the nervous system that shifts the body to a resting, healing mode.

Between each of these breaths, take one normal inhale and exhale—and then begin again. Inhale, filling all the way up to the top with fresh air, and then exhale, making a slight shooshing sound while extending the exhale for as long as possible. Actively push the navel toward the spine in the most controlled manner possible to expel every bit—until there's no air left.

Take a normal breath, and then start again. About three to five of these long, controlled breaths are all you may need to feel a significant change in the body and mindstate.

Tip

Try adding a visualization to increase the benefits of this exercise. To make this breath even more powerful, imagine that on the inhale you are taking in pure energy, pure light, or unlimited potential. See it flowing in and charging the inner body (whatever that looks like for you). On the out-breath you visualize yourself expelling any stagnancy, physical pain, mental stress, emotional turmoil, fatigue, doubt, or confusion. See this leaving the body during the slow exhale—disintegrating and melting into the atmosphere.

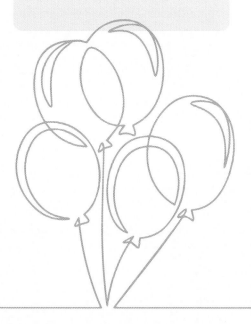

12

Breathing for Physical Release

The exercise combines the breath with a simple visualization. Once you have practiced the full exercise below you can practice miniature check-ins at any time of the day and apply a conscious breath to assist with release of physical symptoms like muscle fatigue or strain, joint pain, headaches, or whatever is ailing you physically.

One-part meditation

Takes 5–10 minutes

Level Beginner

Preparation Find any comfortable seated position on a chair or a cushion on the floor, where the spine can be straight and tall. You can also lie on your back.

Find a comfortable seated position, where the spine can be straight and tall. The shoulders should be encouraged to relax down, the hands should soften. Alternately, lie down on your back and allow the limbs to relax out to the sides.

Begin to watch your breath, noticing the quality of each inhale and each exhale. How does the breath feel coming into your body at this moment?

If the breath feels shallow or limited, are there any simple, small adjustments that can make it feel more expansive and free, such as relaxing the shoulders or softening the abdomen even more? If so, make them now.

Allow the breath to be full and natural as you begin to make the in- and out-breaths an equal length. Gradually slowing everything down. Breathe as slowly as you can comfortably.

Now notice any areas of the body that may feel tense, restricted, fatigued, or even painful. Bring your attention to each of these areas, one by one, and imagine you can send your breath straight into the discomfort. You may want to start at the feet and gently scan the body to the top of the head. Each time you find something that needs attention, send your breath there to do the work.

Get the sense that when you inhale you are creating space and healing where it is needed, and when you exhale you are relieving the body of any residual tension or fatigue. Use your imagination to continue breathing like this—breathe into any areas that need healing and relaxation. And exhale out, allowing all tension to simply melt away.

And continue this process with each area of the body that needs your attention. Imagine strongly that the breath has a healing power. That it creates space for you. Feel the breath massaging the area, sending it the nutrients it needs to heal, stirring the energy around the cells, muscles, nerves, joints, and organs.

Remember that throughout the day you can take short moments to check in, and if you notice any areas of discomfort or irritation, you can consciously send your attention there on the breath, giving that body part, those organs, those tissues, permission to relax, rejuvenate, or heal.

The healing breath
Try to get the strong feeling that the breath is doing all the work that is needed for your particular situation, injury, or discomfort. Slow the breath down and focus it—make it as intentional as possible. In your imagination, see the area receiving the breath in as much detail as possible. Trust that it knows exactly what to do.

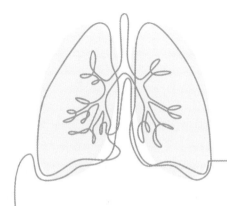

13

Progressive Muscle Relaxation

Progressive muscle relaxation (PMR) techniques have been used for many years by psychologists and doctors alike to alleviate symptoms of stress, physical pain, and insomnia. The conscious attention is rotated around the body, and muscle group or body parts are activated by squeezing the muscles tightly. When these are released a strong sense of relaxation takes over and the entire nervous system benefits.

One-part meditation

Takes 5–10 minutes

Level Beginner

Preparation Lie on your back in bed. When you are treating physical pain or insomnia, then lying down can be the best option.

As you lie back in your bed, take a few moments to get as comfortable as you can. Begin to watch your breath. Feel the slight rise and fall in the belly.

Without trying to change the breath, just let it move naturally as you follow it with your full attention. We'll begin to bring our thoughts inward to the experience of the body so that we can gently encourage and guide it to relax or sleep.

Feel the belly receiving the breath, then softening down again and surrendering. Receiving the life-giving breath and releasing completely once again.

In this exercise we're going to bring our full attention to each part of the body individually—taking a moment to really feel into the area and then to slowly but completely tense the muscles, squeezing them tightly for a count of 10.

When you are releasing the muscles, let the area fully soften and disintegrate, as if it were melting away from your awareness completely.

We'll begin down at the feet. Gently guide your attention down to the left foot and toes.

Now begin to slowly tense the muscles of the left foot and toes. Continue to breathe as you count down from 10:

10-9-8-7-6-5-4-3-2-1

And relax now. Let all the tension sink out of the left foot.

Move to the left lower leg. Begin to contract the muscles of this area, squeezing tightly for:

10-9-8-7-6-5-4-3-2-1

Relax the lower leg completely.

Now the left upper leg and thigh, activating and squeezing tightly for:

10-9-8-7-6-5-4-3-2-1

Releasing all tension in the leg now. Even the most subtle.

The left hip and buttocks area now. Tense and release.

The entire left leg now is sinking down, feeling heavy.

Now bring your attention to the right foot and toes. Tense and activate, counting back from 10.

Release and let go of the right foot completely.

Continue in the same manner with the rest of the body. Each time you release an area, imagine it falling downward. Feel that all tension is gone. That all physical sensation is dissipating.

Move on to the right lower leg, the right upper leg.

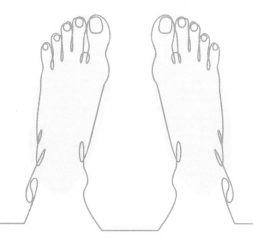

Now turn your attention to the right hip and buttocks region.

Both legs are now completely heavy and releasing downward.

Come to the left hand and fingers, then the left forearm, before moving on to the left upper arm and shoulder.

Come now to the right hand and fingers, then the right forearm, before moving on to the right upper arm and shoulder.

Both arms are now completely relaxed, melting away from the torso.

Now turn to the muscles of the entire back, all the way up and down the spine, tensing, activating, and energizing.

Move to the abdomen and chest area, then the neck and throat.

And now move to the muscles of the face, the head, and scalp. Soften and release, so there's no expression left on the face.

Feel your entire body opening and softening, becoming heavier and heavier.

There is no more movement, just stillness, peace, and quiet as the body drops into a deep, healing, receptive state.

Surrender the body over to a deep rest. Invite the body to be repaired and rejuvenated, as you rest.

Invite the conscious mind to give way to the subconscious mind.

Let deep relaxation slowly wash over the body. Warm and soft. Everything is dissolving and letting go now. Release.

Tip

A particular order of body relaxation is not required, but try to do the limbs first and the head and face last. You can pair body parts for a shorter practice—like both feet and then both lower legs, etc. If an area seems challenging to squeeze and activate physically without moving the body much, just do your best and imagine everything tensing there. Imagine that each layer of muscle is responding to your attention.

14

Affirming Serenity

The internal self-talk that is perpetually active in our minds influences everything about our lives. Studies have shown that affirmations activate parts of the reward center of the brain, which may give us a feeling of satisfaction and satiation, as well as the part of the control center that deals with self-referential information. This is the area of the brain that writes and tells the stories of who we are in this world—of what we expect and desire and what we deeply believe about ourselves and the world around us. Affirmation work can help to shift and rewrite our story about what we believe to be ultimately true, so we can have a more open mind and begin to actively create the life and experiences we most want.

One-part meditation

Takes 5–20 minutes

Level Beginner

Preparation Find any comfortable seated position on a chair or a cushion on the floor. You can also lie on your back or stand.

Begin by finding a comfortable seat, or lie on your back or stand up. Allow the body to be alert, yet relaxed and comfortable.

Bring your attention to your breath, without trying to change it. Just notice the condition or state of the breath right now. How does it feel? With a slight curiosity of mind, what qualities do you find in your own breath, in this moment?

Now, with your attention resting on each inhale and exhale, gradually begin to slow your breath down. Make the inhales and exhales an equal length. Feel the breath softening and slowing.

Allow your lower abdomen to soften and round out—receiving each in-breath fully. And when you exhale, allow any stress or fatigue to roll off of the physical body. Take as many conscious breaths as you need to fully release it.

Now, to increase the benefits of the slow, rhythmic breath, we'll start to add an affirmation to each inhale and exhale. Let the spirit of the message influence you if it will. Try not to think about the meaning of the affirmation or define what it may mean in any particular circumstance. Just repeat it with faith and witness your body's response.

Let's begin with the affirmation: "I am calm."

On your inhale, mentally repeat: "I am."

On your exhale, mentally repeat: "Calm." Inhale "I am," then exhale "calm."

I am—calm.
I am—calm.

Continue on, listening to the words mindfully as they synchronize with the breath. It's almost as if they occur there naturally. Once the message feels clear and comforting, and your body and mind seem to be embracing it, move on to the next affirmation.

Next, on the inhale, repeat to yourself "I am" but exhale "at peace." Inhaling "I am," then exhaling "at peace."

I am—at peace.
I am—at peace.

Keep going with each affirmation for as long as feels right to you, today.

Now inhaling "I am" and exhaling "safe."

I am—safe.
I am—safe.

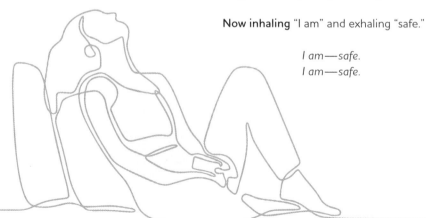

When you're ready, allow the affirmations to simply fade away with your next exhale, and return your fullest attention to the breath. Notice the sensation, the movement of this life energy, flowing in and out now.

Now leave the breath as it is, and notice the body. How does the body feel? What qualities can you observe in it?

Remember that you can always return to this state at any point in time by simply listening for one or all of those affirmations, occurring naturally and traveling through the body on the breath.

When you're ready, allow your eyes to open softly. Take a moment to enjoy this feeling.

The more you practice this exercise, the more you will synch your body, mind, and emotions, and create a powerful memory of calm and relaxation that you can return to over and over, just by using your positive attention.

With gratitude, acknowledge the time you've taken for yourself.

The more you practice positive affirmations—even by threading them into daily activities—the more quickly and easily you'll be able to return to this balanced, harmonious state of being at will.

Repeating affirmations

When first getting familiar with a meditative practice of affirmative self-talk, be especially compassionate to yourself and try to keep a very open mind. If there is strong resistance to a particular phrase, then skip that one for now (but maybe stay open to revisiting it in the future). Listen for the feeling that is transmitted by the words rather than focusing on their intellectual meaning. Begin by practicing the example phrases given here, but then feel free to create some positive affirmations of your own. Write them down and practice the formal exercise with them, or set reminders (in your phone or on a stickie note) to take a few moments from your normal routine to check in and repeat your favorite one on your breath a few times.

15

Ocean Breath

This breathing technique creates a slight sound on the inhale and the exhale that is used as a meditative focus. The practitioner gently constricts the passage of the air at the back of the throat so that a very soft hissing noise is produced. Attention is placed on the noise vibration and this is controlled gently. Then it can be used to relax and steady the mind, and create internal focus.

One-part meditation

Takes 5–20 minutes

Level Beginner to Intermediate

Preparation Find any comfortable seated position on a chair or a cushion on the floor.

Once you're sitting comfortably, begin by steadying the breath. Bring your inhales and exhales to an equal length, and start counting to 6 for each breath in and to 6 for each breath out.

In this exercise, we'll practice developing a very soft ocean breath by closing the back of the throat *just* slightly so as to constrict the passage of air. This friction will create a very quiet sound, something like a sigh or gentle white noise. You may only be able to hear it internally, or it may be slightly audible, and either is okay. But it should feel comfortable, without any sense of strain. Try to keep the sound as consistent and steady as possible on both the in- and out-breaths.

Go ahead now and give it a try. Close the back of the throat just enough to achieve a steady air sound on each breath. Continue your 6 count breaths, but pay attention to the sensation of the air— now more acute, passing through the throat and nose. Pay particular attention to the sound and its qualities. It may even be more subtle on the inhale than the exhale, but the sound is always present. The belly is soft and air is flowing down where it will, comfortably.

If it helps your mind to relax, you can imagine the sound as waves coming in and going back out to sea. Or, if you prefer, see the sound as calming white noise, drowning out all persistent thoughts and concerns for the time-being and soothing your system. Feel the soft vibration of the breath occurring through the lungs, throat, nose, and all of the connected muscles and organs.

Tip
For this version of ocean breath (also called ujjayi breathing in yoga), the volume is very soft and the breath stays subtle. You should be able to sense the friction and vibration somewhere in the throat without any discomfort or strain. Experiment with the amount of air to find the most relaxing version of this for you at any given time.

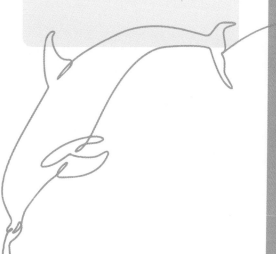

16

Belly Breathing

In this exercise we're going to use the diaphragm, the largest breathing muscle, to extend and deepen the breath and to attain smooth control of both inhales and exhales. When the abdomen is relaxed the diaphragm can move downward from under the ribs and create a gentle massaging pressure to soothe the internal organs, assisting with healthy digestion and elimination. This action also helps stimulate the vagus nerve which sends a message to the brain to turn on the parasympathetic Rest and Digest nervous system. The reflexive response from the brain reduces heart rate, circulating stress hormones, and blood pressure, and prepares the body for deep, healing rest and repair.

Two-part meditation

Takes 5 minutes

Level Beginner

Preparation Find a comfortable position lying on the floor, on cushions, or on a bed—just make sure you're fully supported, whether that means propping up your knees so they're slightly bent to relax the lower back and soften the abdomen, or supporting the head and neck with a small pillow.

Part 1

Allow the spine to lengthen gently and the legs to relax completely, rolling outward. Let the chest be broad with the arms positioned away from the body, palms facing up. Take a few moments here to feel the weight of the body sinking down. Relaxing all of the points of contact or pressure into the floor or bed. Notice and then relax the contact points one by one. And then notice them all at once and see them release simultaneously.

Begin to shift your focus to your breath— just watching the natural flow, in and out. Start to notice where the breath is moving now. Where is the air flowing most easily inside the body at this moment in time?

In this exercise, we'll imagine there is a balloon in the lower abdomen and that with each inhale you are fully filling the balloon up—slowly but surely rounding out the belly so that it can receive all the air. Then, with each exhale, you'll slowly let that air retreat and leave the body, deflating the balloon little by little—smoothly and consistently. From the time the air enters the nostrils to the time the belly is full, you'll count mentally to 10. The pace will feel different for each individual, but there should be no strain or discomfort—just inhale for 10 counts.

Let's begin. Counting to yourself now, inhale to 10 through the nose and right down into the base of the belly. Gently direct the air into the lowest abdominal region. Fill all the way up without forcing.

Now exhale, smoothly and consistently, for a count of 10. Allow the abdomen to soften back down and the navel to just fall back toward the spine. The lowest part of the abdomen emptying first. When the inhale comes again, fill the lowest part of the body. And then allow the belly to soften and relax as the air floats out continuously again.

Continue breathing in this way, trying to even the breath out using gentle, but focused, muscular control. Think about your diaphragm—the muscle underneath the bottom ribs, just under the lungs. Imagine what it looks like as it expands and pushes down as you inhale, creating suction for the air to flow in naturally. And then, with control, see this large muscle receding back up underneath the bottom ribs as it releases—increasing the pressure in the abdominothoracic region so that the air is expelled naturally.

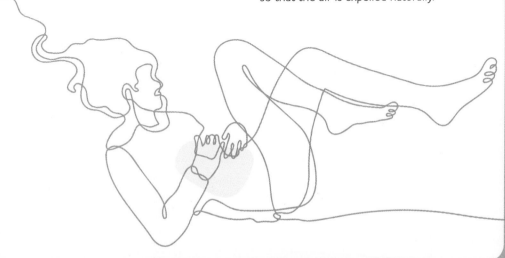

Continue breathing through the nose with control to fill up the belly. Deep, steady, but comfortable breaths. Then slowly and smoothly release the air from the belly up and out through the nose.

Continue on like this for a couple more minutes—visualizing using the diaphragm muscle to assist the smoothness of your breathing and even to help massage the adjacent internal organs. If your mind wanders off with thought or other body sensations, just notice where it went and ever so gently bring the mind back to the counting and the physical experience of this breath.

Gradually now let this breath fade away—slowly. Let the breath return to normal and watch the natural breath now, as it enters and exits by itself.

Take a few moments to notice how you feel and give yourself thanks for the experience. When you come to sit or stand up, move slowly and make sure to feel steady.

Part 2

Make sure you're comfortable enough that you can completely let the body soften down. Legs relax out to the side, arms away from the body slightly with the palms up, and neck long. Feel the body really heavying down. Begin to notice the weight of the body, and all of the points of pressure. Where is the body in contact with the floor, the bed? As you notice these points of contact, let them melt down and release even more.

And softly bring your attention to the breath. Not changing it yet, just watching the natural in- and out-breaths—noticing the way they move, the way they feel right now. Notice where in the body the breath is reaching. Make a mental map of your breath. Without changing anything right now—just notice if the breath is traveling to every possible space, every suitable location. Are you able to breathe easily at your maximum capacity? Or are parts shut down or restricted? What does the breathing look like, right now?

In this exercise, we're going to practice three-part breathing by directing the breath, using the diaphragm muscle. The three parts are the belly, the center of the chest, and the uppermost part of the chest/base of the throat. Create a mental image of those three sections. In this version of diaphragmatic breathing, we'll inhale in this pattern and we'll also exhale in this pattern—from the bottom (belly) to the top (uppermost chest/ throat). We usually have the most air capacity and movement in the middle section of the chest and the least in the uppermost chest and base of the throat. That's normal, and there's no need to try to make the parts equal. It's only important to bring attention to them in the correct order, from bottom to top, every time the breath moves.

To help you imagine the three parts more clearly, and physically feel their movement, you can place one hand on the belly, so the palm is resting on the navel, and the other hand on the chest—the palm should be right at the center of the chest over the breastbone and the thumb should touch near the base of the throat, where the sternum meets the clavicle, or collarbone. This will help you to sense the air entering and expanding all three of these areas, independently.

Let's begin. Very, very slowly inhale through the nose, down into the very lowest part of the belly. Feel it expanding and feel the hand placed there raising upward. Now fill the midsection of the chest and rib cage, the breath now pressing the palm of your other hand upward and the ribs out to the sides. And, finally, more subtly, filling the very top section where the thumb is resting.

Very slowly exhale from the nose, emptying from the base of the belly first and letting the hand follow the navel as it sinks toward the spine. Then from the chest, emptying the air slowly. And, finally, the last drop of air from the base of the throat and breastbone area.

Again, inhaling down into a rounding belly, and then into the midsection as the lungs inflate, and then into the top. Exhaling out from the belly, navel falling back, from the rib cage and middle of the chest, and any air left in the top of the chest and throat, gently escaping.

Continue like this, watching the rising and falling in these three distinct sections. Allow the breath to be slow, but natural. No force and no strain. Explore what it feels like to access each of these areas independently with your breath.

How have the sensations of the breath shifted, now that you're consciously directing it, with control, in this manner?

Very gradually now, begin to let those three distinct sections meld together, little by little. Let the borders that define them begin to soften and fade away. Still breathing from the base to the top, base to the top, allow the breath to undulate, to become more easy, more fluid.

Completely dissolve the boundaries between the three sections now, and continue to witness the breath. Is the breath moving differently now? Can you notice the feeling of the breath in the back-body now—pressing into the support? Or in any other areas that it may not have been flowing freely to in the beginning?

Let the breath return to normal and come back to its natural pace. Stay here with this for a few more minutes—observing, sensing, noticing any differences at all in the breath, body, and mindstate.

When you're ready, start to feel the weight of the body once more. Notice the body and where it is in space. Feel the bones, the muscles, the skin. Feel the face. Take a deep breath in, and when you exhale allow your eyes to flutter open softly. If you move to sit or stand up, then move slowly.

Tip

Slowing the breath down allows the mind to relax and signals to cells that it's time to heal and repair, that it's time to detoxify and clean out—both physically and energetically.

When we learn to control the breath, we can more easily control the body and mind. Like other forms of diaphragmatic breathing, this exercise helps strengthen and refine the breathing muscles, which can be very therapeutic for the digestive and respiratory systems, among others. It also helps create a deep state of relaxation where stress can begin to melt away—the physical, mental, and chemical components of excess stress are allowed to dissolve.

17

Countdown to Sleep

The simple act of counting can give a busy mind something to focus on. Counting is one of the first things we master when we begin to learn a language, and it is so deeply ingrained that it becomes second nature. If we can focus on counting without overthinking, before long the thoughts settle, emotions calm, and the physical body can follow suit and release into a rejuvenating sleep.

One-part meditation

Takes 10 minutes

Level Beginner

Preparation Lie in bed on your back, and prepare for sleep. Make yourself as comfortable as possible with pillows, blankets, and anything else that relaxes you, and prepare yourself for a long, deep sleep.

As you lie down to rest in that comfortable and safe place, your bed, allow your body to soften down and let all of your muscles relax and loosen. Feel them getting heavier—releasing.

Notice the breath, softly rising and falling in the belly and chest. Place one palm on the body to help focus your attention on this rising-falling movement. Know that sleep is coming naturally. It's already on the way.

Start to release any physical fatigue or any sensations of discomfort that may still remain in the body—on every single exhale, let go even more. Inhale, and notice the belly lifting up. Exhale, seeing any tension draining away.

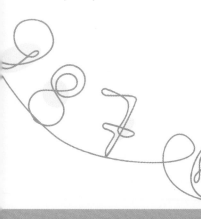

The breath is natural and gentle. And it continues with this process—lifting gently and then letting everything go. There's nothing more to do. Nothing more to figure out. Nothing left but to just rest and release into a deep, healing sleep. Any questions and concerns from the day that may still be clinging are no longer valid here. You'll approach them again tomorrow, in a new form—feeling recharged, rested, and confident. Clear and bright and balanced.

On your exhales now, imagine any remaining thoughts or concerns in the mind simply melting out of the body, down through the bed, and back into the earth. Inhale, belly rises. Exhale, any mental strain is freed.

In a moment, we'll begin to count the breaths. On each exhale, noting the breath, moving downward from 100. During the countdown, if there's anything left in the body or the mind that needs to be released, surrender it and allow it to let go with each out-breath.

Let's begin now, inhaling... and exhaling from 100:

> Inhaling... and exhaling 99...
> Inhaling ... and exhaling 98...

Continue on your own, at a natural pace. If you forget what number you are on, don't be concerned. Just start again at 100, and continue counting the out-breaths all the way down to 1.

The belly rises softly, and simply falls back down. Feel this gentle rhythm like waves coming in to shore and back out to sea. At some point, you will surrender the body and mind over to deep sleep.

With every breath comes quietude. With every breath comes tranquility. Serenity. With every breath you release more and more into the bed. Let go. And receive deep, healing rest.

Tip
If the task of counting down from 100 feels too mentally stimulating, try starting this exercise at 50 or even 20 and simply repeat when you arrive at 1. The goal is for the counting down to feel quite simple, but not completely effortless—the subtle focus required is key to the relaxation effect.

18

Easy Sleep

When the body is in a deep sleep all muscles are completely soft and the heart rate and breathing become slow. By imitating a deep-sleep stage—relaxing the muscles and slowing the breath, heart, and brain waves using meditation—we can artificially stimulate the same physiological effects of deep-sleep stages, triggering the nervous system to fall into a deep night's sleep much faster.

One-part meditation

Takes 10 minutes

Level Beginner

Preparation Lie in bed on your back, and make yourself as comfortable as possible with pillows, blankets, and anything else to prepare you for a good night's sleep (lavender essential oil, an eye cover, etc).

Begin to relax more deeply now, little by little letting the layers of stress and overthinking fall away. Notice the points of pressure between the body and the surface of the bed.

Notice the weight of the body and the feeling of the pillows and the covers caressing you. Know that you're supported and safe. It's that time to let go of any body tension, of any physical stress or fatigue, and hand the body over to deep, rejuvenating sleep.

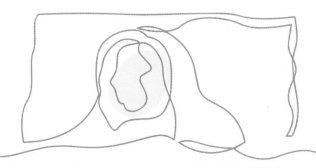

It's that time to let go of any persistent thoughts, questions, worries, or concerns. And hand the mind and body over to deep, renewing sleep. Know that with each breath in this calm place, your body is becoming softer. Your heart rate is slowing down. And your muscles are releasing. Your brain is starting to let go of unnecessary activity or energy.

All of your being seems to be becoming more and more spacious—full of soft, radiant light. You're becoming receptive, returning to your natural state. You're preparing for deep sleep that will recharge you overnight, and reignite your vital life force upon awakening.

Feel all of the components of the body now, as if they were exhaling a slow sigh... Sense the relief that comes with allowing them to let go and receive profound rest and nurturing.

As the breath continues to slow down, becoming a bit more shallow, yet consistent and steady, start to notice that all the sensation of the physical body is dissipating, dissolving completely. See yourself relaxing so thoroughly that you lose all body sensation. There's nowhere to go, nothing left to do. Just allow the body and mind to sink into a deep and complete healing rest.

Tip
Autosuggestions like the ones below are subconscious directives that can help you relax, surrender, and drop into deep sleep. Try creating a few of your own, and repeat them as many times as it feels good. See yourself planting them in your subconscious so that they can blossom as reminders during your rest.

If you feel any resistance, you can tell your body and mind that:

It's okay to let go now.
I allow myself deep rest.
I am ready to start again.
I am safe.

Know that as you slumber you will continue to release all discomfort or tension as the body and mind return naturally to a relaxed and balanced state.

19

Guided Sleep Relaxation

This exercise is focused on releasing as much physical tension and stress from the body as possible before sleep (and often at the beginning of a savasana pose in yoga), so you can more quickly access deep, healing sleep states. You'll move your attention to each body part and then imagine it warming, melting, and immediately releasing.

One-part meditation

Takes 10 minutes

Level Beginner

Preparation Lie in bed on your back, and prepare for deep sleep by supporting yourself with pillows, blankets, and anything that helps you to relax and feel comfortable (lavender essential oil, an eye cover, etc).

Rest back fully into the bed and allow the body to become heavier. See the muscles softening. Let everything begin to melt down. It's time to allow the body to slip away into deep relaxation. Notice how even the breath is slowing down now, all by itself.

Now bring your awareness all the way down to the left foot. With your attention strongly engaged, ask the toes to relax, one by one. See each of them soften and release. See the left foot—the sole and the top of the foot. Place all of your attention there, flooding the whole area and everything in between. Relax the left foot. All fatigue and tension melting out. Bring your focus now to the left ankle. Relax the ankle, all the way through, letting go of any discomfort or sensations. Now the left lower leg and calf. The muscles melting away from the bone, completely and totally relaxed. The left knee. From front to back and to each side, and all the way through the joint, see every structure softening and warming in the knee. Relax. Move to the left upper leg and thigh. Feel it becoming heavier, softening and surrendering down— release. The left hip, all the way around to the seat. Everything warming, sinking down heavy. Relax even more now.

Move the attention now down to the right foot and toes. Begin by relaxing the toes, one by one. Softening, warming,

releasing. Relax the sole and the top of the foot, and everything in between. Moving the attention to the right ankle— seeing everything there let go. The right lower leg and calf—warming and melting down. Release all tension. The right knee—all the way through, seeing lots of space inside to release. The right thigh and upper leg—muscles, nerves, bones— sinking down heavy. Release. The right hip, all the way through to the seat— everything melting down. Soft and heavy.

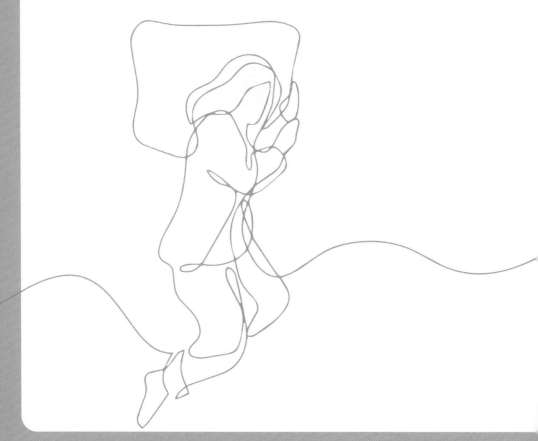

Move your attention to the lower back and spine. Visualize lots of space between the vertebrae—muscles and nerves relaxing away from the bones. Warm and heavy. Release the lower back. The middle back and spine now. Allow them to feel spacious and free. Broadening and sinking down—very heavy. Relax. The upper back, spine, and shoulder blades. All layers releasing, one by one. Heaving down, tension draining away. Relax.

Bring your attention to the abdomen. See it warming, softening, sinking down. The solar plexus area—surrendering, giving way to warm, gentle sensation. The chest and rib cage—soft, light, and free. Feel a sense of openness as the muscles of the front body relax down and back.

Move your attention now to the left hand and fingertips. Relax the fingers, letting them unfold and soften down with the palm melting open. No more sense of grasping. Just the freedom of letting go. The left forearm—all the muscles melting away. Dissolving. The left elbow and upper arm—heavy, sinking away from the body. Relax. The right hand and fingertips. Melting open, soft and loose. Release the right forearm now—muscles melting away from bone. The right elbow and upper arm—sinking down, tension disappearing.

Both shoulders rolling back and sinking down deeply. Release. The neck and throat—all tension draining away. Feel the entire area warm and supple, melting down further. Soften the jaw, the area around the mouth, cheeks, and nose, and relax the area around the eyes and temples. Let the forehead and scalp warm and melt back even further now. Relax.

Now visualize all of the internal organs resting. Peacefully sinking back. Visualize everything working perfectly. Relax.

You are free now to leave the body all by itself. All sensation gone. All perception dimming. Trust that every part of you is resting and healing itself perfectly while you drift away into a deep, renewing sleep.

Tip

Try pairing this guided relaxation with soft, calming music or a natural soundscape that can play at a low level, uninterrupted in the background while you sleep. Really try to feel the depth of the relaxation in each part. If you like, you can visualize a place or time when your body and muscles feel exceptionally relaxed—in a hot jacuzzi bath, pressing into warm sand on the beach, having a massage, or any other scene where your physical body quickly responds and lets go.

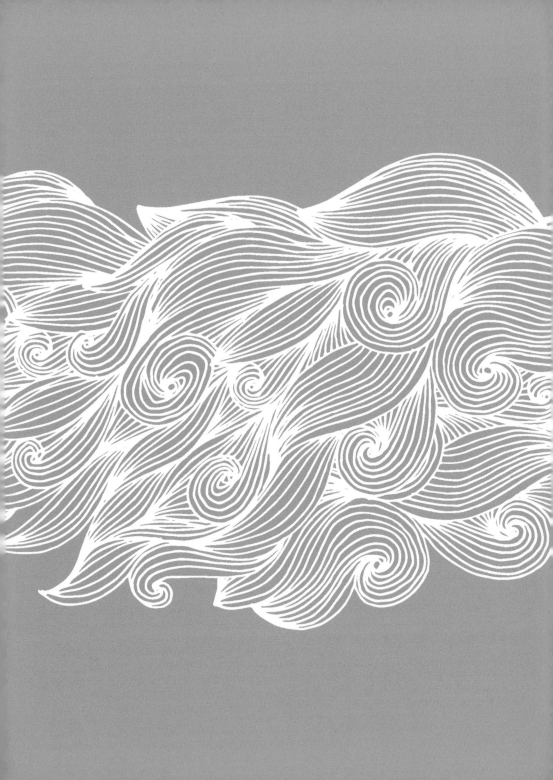

CHAPTER 3
VISUALIZE

Visualization is a technique used in meditation practice to focus the mind on a particular subject matter. With practice and dedication, we can learn to keep returning to the thoughts that we consciously choose to see and experience, rather than ones that may be unhelpful and insignificant. Eventually, we can stay longer with the thoughts that make us feel good and bring excitement, and devote more of our attention to them. You can make anything stronger by bringing your attention to it.

Visualization

Although we don't all visualize in the same way, if we use meditation to improve our concentration and sensitivity we can all find the feeling-place of our thoughts. We all have the ability to choose certain thoughts, focus on them, and let the feeling of those thoughts wash over us. Sometimes it's easy to sink into a daydream and visualize all of the details until you really feel like you're right there, and other times the mind is distracted and we have to keep rebuilding the image in the mind and trying to "feel into" it.

One key to successful visualization is focusing on the details. Try to see what it is you're imagining in as much detail as possible. You'll know you're going in the right direction when the details you imagine continue to feel good and seem to produce a sense of excitement, joy, peace, or even quiet calm in your body. Notice how your body actually feels when you are thinking about your vision or goal—and keep moving steadily toward those particular details that produce positive feelings.

If you feel any negativity toward your own visualization—if you feel, for example, that you don't really deserve it, could never really have it, or that it just would never actually happen for you—be patient and mindful. Acknowledge that you're hitting some resistance. Resistance is normal at the beginning of this type of practice, so don't let it discourage you. Just keep practicing the meditations that resonate with you, and when you come to visualize a goal or an outcome, be easy with it. Back off of any detail that casts doubt and go more general for a few moments. Find the feeling-place of excitement or peacefulness by making your vision less grandiose, less detailed for now. Back up a bit and work on something that you really believe is attainable at some point in the near future. Start small and make increasing gains—just as you would when strengthening any muscle in the body.

Resistance is normal at the beginning of this type of practice, so don't let it discourage you.

With a visualization practice you are training the mind to feel good by triggering the feeling of getting what you want. Start with a small goal or desire and gradually work your way up as your comfort and confidence increases. You're rebuilding your inner structure and belief system and reuniting with your inner being, inner child, guardian spirit—or whatever you may call it. Everyone is born deserving of happiness and abundance. Through visualization and meditation, we can begin to see how on track we are with truly acknowledging and accepting this for ourselves, and we can begin to have some conscious control over what we attract and allow into our lives.

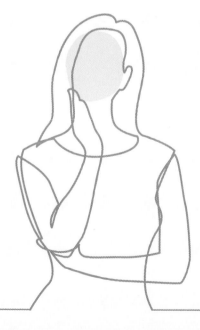

20

Energy Boost

This exercise can bring a fresh charge of energy to both the mind and the body in only a few short minutes. It's similar to the calming Ocean Breath exercise in that the back of the throat is gently contracted, but this time the breath and sound are more vigorous and rapid. If you feel light-headed or dizzy at any point in this exercise, stop and breathe normally. Begin with short amounts of time and increase if your body responds positively.

One-part meditation

Takes 2–5 minutes

Level Beginner

Preparation Sit in an upright position where the spine can be straight and the breath full and free in its movement. Lift your chest a little and bring the shoulders down and back. Make the back of the neck long and soften the belly. You should feel alert, yet relaxed.

Begin by tuning into the breath and bringing all of your awareness to whatever place in the body you feel the breath most acutely right now. This could be at the tip of the nose or just inside the nostrils, at the center of the chest causing a rising and falling movement, in the belly, expanding and relaxing again. Or anywhere else that you feel the breath most strongly. Now see if you can accentuate the sensation happening at that most vivid point. Can you make the sensation a little bit more noticeable? Can you pull a bit more air in at the nostrils, lift the chest higher or wider, or soften the belly to receive more air there? Can you make your awareness more keen?

Now begin to close the back of the throat just slightly, so that the breath makes a soft noise (like the Ocean Breath exercise, but more audible). Watch the waves going in and going back out. Create just a slight restriction there at the back of the throat so that a vibration is produced internally, like energizing white noise. Try to equalize both the length and force of the in- and out-breaths.

Continue to accentuate on the inhale, gradually deepening the expansion and sensation. Making every breath more audible. Then, on the exhale, use the abdominal muscles to push the navel toward the spine, gently but firmly expelling all of the air back out.

Begin to breathe just a little bit faster and just a little bit stronger now. Inhaling for 3 counts now and exhaling for 3 counts. Always breathing through the nose, but still making noise as the air passes through the contracted upper chest and throat.

Inhale, lift, and expand even more than usual for 3 counts. Exhale using the abdominal muscles to press the air from the belly for 3 counts. Continue like this, paying attention to the friction and vibration at the back of the throat, almost as if you're sipping the air in through a straw. Fill up every tiny space you can find in the chest, rib cage, back, and side-bodies. Imagine you can energize your entire being with the breath energy, make all of the cells more alert and more awake.

Every time you exhale, there's even more space for fresh energy. Every time you inhale, watch a new, responsive breath moving into any areas of the body that need to be invigorated. Anything that's feeling fatigued or tired is getting a high dose of energy straight from your breath now.

With the last couple of breaths, visualize yourself directly charging any place else in the body that needs a little energy. And then let your breath just come back to normal. Watch the breath as it settles into its natural rhythm. Take notice of the physical body—does it feel any different now? Notice your face, your hands and feet, your arms and legs, your midsection, the top of the head. Is your posture a little taller and straighter? And noticing your normal breath now—how does it feel?

Notice this energized state—this new alertness of all of the cells, all of the tissues. A focused awareness of the muscles or organs. Maybe a slight tingling, effervescent sensation across the skin and face. A new-found mental sharpness.

Open your eyes, remembering that any time you need to enhance your energy—mental or physical—you can take a few moments to concentrate on the breath like this, charging and energizing any place you bring your attention to.

21

Dissolve Mental Stress

This exercise was created to address headaches—all types of tension headaches, migraines, and referred pain. It can also be used to soften and loosen any negative thoughts or thought patterns that you may have become aware of during your meditation practice, such as negativity, rumination, self-judgment, and anything that may feel like an irritant to the mind and head space.

One-part meditation

Takes 15–20 minutes

Level Beginner

Preparation Find any position that feels supportive and comfortable, whether that is sitting up in a chair or on a cushion on the floor, or lying on your back. Let the spine lengthen so it's relatively straight and alleviated of extra pressure. Take care to position your neck and head so they can be as relaxed as possible.

Notice your breath, as it is right now. Just watch its natural ebb and flow, the natural in-and-out rhythm. Pay attention to any sensations that arise on the breath for the next few moments.

Begin to slow the breath down gently now—just a tad, gradually. Take notice of the weight of your seat in the chair or on the floor, or your back where it's contacting the floor or bed. Feel them becoming a little heavier. Grounding you. Securing you.

Now gently move your awareness to the head. Take a moment to notice any sensations around the head, skull, and scalp. Now imagine you can gaze inward, without reacting to any perceptions you may or may not have—just looking and discovering, and curiously assessing what you sense. Where are the sensations coming from? Are they concentrated in one area?

Imagine any areas of the head that feel blocked, tight, or painful as being filled with compact sand. Billions of granules of sand all pressed together, taking up space. Creating the sensation of intense pressure. The sharp edges of the granules creating irritation and discomfort.

Now channel your imagination and see a pure, continuous stream of cool water begin to flow, entering the top center of the head and flowing straight out through the bottom of the feet. A tap is turned on above you, and this steady and powerful and tenacious stream of cleansing water flows. As the water flows through you, it is breaking apart the sand formations—dissolving them, melting them, and slowly flushing the granules down toward the feet and out of the body—little by little by little. Feel the sensation of relief.

Continue this process, really imagining you can see any areas of discomfort softening and giving way to the steady flow of water. Feel the sensation of the water purifying everything it touches, and the power and force inherent in it, which changes the landscape just as it does on the Earth's surface, to create space and form a new shape. Let every last granule of sand exit the body this way, out through the feet, back to the Earth.

Allow the water to continue to flow into the top of the head, but now just cooling and soothing any remaining stress or fatigue in the head and the body. Feel it now purifying, renewing, recharging your brain and mind.

When this process feels complete for you, simply release the visualization and bring yourself back to the sensation of the breath. Begin to inhale several times, imagining the breath moving from the base of the spine to the top of the head and back down. Notice with all of your senses the feeling of balance and clarity that now exists where there was once a blockage. The next time you inhale up to the top of the head, release the exhale from that same place—at the top of the head—allowing it to flow up and outward, freeing any pressure that may remain.

Allow your eyes to open gently. Take a moment to recognize the shift that your attention has brought to your condition, and to appreciate taking the time to explore your innate power of healing.

The power of water

Water is used as an aid to visualization because it has the distinctive power of transformation. In nature, water dilutes, purifies, dissolves, carves, and shapes everything that it touches.

22

Heart Health

This exercise brings healing energy and attention to both your physical heart and its connections and to your energetic or emotional heart center. In Eastern medicine these exist in the same area, and have overlapping functions. This meditation focuses on relieving stress and anxiety from the physical architecture of the heart and its components, and also on harmonizing energetic aspects of creating receptivity and compassion for yourself and others.

One-part meditation

Takes 15–20 minutes

Level Beginner

Preparation Find a comfortable position in a chair or lying on your back, preferably in a quiet space that you find relaxing. Let the spine be straight, yet supple, and the body relaxed, yet alert. Position yourself so that your heart center can feel supported and expansive.

Relax into your meditation posture and begin to slow the breath down just a little. Notice what the breath feels like right now, and how it moves in the chest, side-body, and back.

Now guide your attention down to your feet—place every bit of your focus down at the feet and direct any discomfort or tension there to release now. Very slowly begin to move your awareness upward—smoothly and softly turning your focus to each part of the body, one by one. And wherever you feel tension, anxious movement, vibration, or pain, simply allow that discomfort to dissolve immediately.

Moving on and upward, not spending too much time in any particular place, but fully releasing and relaxing as you go—all the way up to the top of the head.

And when you reach the top of the head, relax your attention down onto your breath near the center of the chest. Feel the small movement there from the waves of breath coming in and out. Whether they're steady or irregular, fast or slow, shallow or deep, it makes no difference. Just notice how your breath is moving right now, maintaining compassion for yourself and a nonjudgmental attitude.

Now start to slow the breath down, very gradually making the inhales and the exhales just a bit longer, and matching their length. Begin counting to 4 as you breathe in and 4 as you breathe out.

Try to rest your full attention on any sensations that come with the breath. Notice how the inhale or the exhale may feel different from one another. Become aware of any sensations at all that may appear in the chest area, the throat, the abdomen, the shoulders, or anywhere else in the body.

Continue breathing in this way, and, if it feels comfortable now, increase the count by 1. Begin inhaling for 5 and then exhaling for 5.

Stay sensitive and notice the intricate qualities that arise while you become familiar with your own breath. Remain calmly alert and also watch the body's reaction to this breath, as it slows and equalizes. While practicing this exercise, there should be no discomfort. So if you feel any sort of strain or irritation, simply take shorter, milder breaths.

Now we're going to begin to count the heartbeats. Your natural heartbeats will guide your counts from now on. On the inhale, count each heartbeat beating 1-2-3-4-5. On the exhale, beating 1-2-3-4-5. Do you notice that your heartbeat is a tiny bit slower on your exhale than your inhale? Continue on like this.

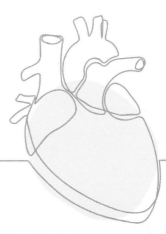

Keep watching the subtleties of the breath, and counting the same number of heartbeats on the in- and out-breaths—even if the exhale begins to become slightly longer than the inhale. You can always use your inner intelligence to increase or decrease the number of counts to what feels most appropriate for you today, in this moment. Keep in mind that the breath should still feel comfortable and natural. If you notice any tension in the physical body—the abdomen, the shoulders, the face or jaw—let it release again and bring your focus right back to the breath and heartbeats.

Now, with your next exhale, simply release the counting and let your breath come back to its natural, normal rhythm. Notice the relaxed sensation—what does it feel like to you? Softness? Warmth? Tingling? Balance?

Now visualize your heart, resting there in your chest. Place your palm or palms over the chest to connect if you wish. See the physical heart relaxed and healthy, calmly pumping to its own perfect rhythm, moving just the right amount of blood through the arteries. All of the blood vessels are healthy, receptive, and responding perfectly to it. See this whole system throughout the body, functioning perfectly now. Visualize it. See it as healthy, clean, vibrant, and strong.

Rest in the knowledge that the body always knows how to heal and take care of itself at its innermost, cellular level. When you train your attention upon the healthy functioning of the heart and blood vessels, you are promoting even more of this innate healing to take place, which carries over long after the exercise ends.

Notice the breath again in the center of the chest now—rising and falling slowly... Notice the weight of the body on the support. And, when you feel ready, let your eyes open and return to the room. Take a moment to acknowledge the time you've committed to encouraging your own inner healing.

Health benefits
Research has shown that the stress-reducing effects of meditation can help curb heart disease, lower blood pressure, reduce stress hormones, and improve the health of heart vessels and cellular tissue.

23

Immunity Boost

In today's global society, the body must defend itself on a daily basis—for example, against foreign invaders like bacteria and viruses, as well as chemicals and environmental pollution. We also know that physical and mental stress can greatly affect the functioning of the immune system and that modern life can expose us collectively to an unprecedented amount of persistent stress. This meditation reduces stress and focuses on allowing the immune system to balance, reboot, and gain strength and accuracy.

One-part meditation

Takes 15–20 minutes

Level Beginner

Preparation Make yourself comfortable lying on your back if possible; otherwise, find a comfortable seated position in a chair or on a cushion on the floor. Let your spine lengthen up slightly as your body grounds down.

Relax into this comfortable position but maintain a gentle alertness. Bring your attention to your breath for a moment, feeling its movement in the body. Feeling it rise and fall in the chest or abdomen. You may notice the breath starting to respond to your attention, gradually slowing down.

Now bring your attention to your feet. Take a moment and notice any sensations that are present there. Then move your attention to the ankles and notice what they feel like right now. And then to the lower legs... The knees... And continuing on slowly until you arrive at the head. Take your time, there is no rush. Notice any feelings, any physical sensations, any information that's available in each part as you bring your full awareness to it. Without judging, without staying anywhere too long or skipping any part completely—just mindfully glide your attention all the way up.

Take note of each area and how it feels right now in this time and place. If you notice anything particularly uncomfortable as you go along, you may want to pause momentarily and ask it to release before you move on to the next part. When you finally arrive at the head, just rest your attention there loosely at the top.

Now imagine a bright white glowing light coming down through the top of the head. See this light illuminating your brain and stimulating its connections and communication with the body's immune

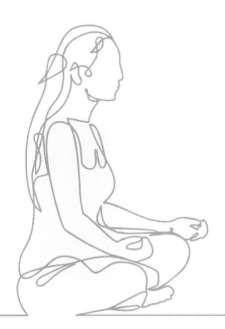

system—calling it to action. The entire skull and brain are now saturated with this vibrant light.

Envision this light traveling down from the brain into the rest of the body—down into the chest, the arms, the torso. Filling each area up completely. Down to the pelvis, the hips, the legs. Seeping into every tiny space and lighting it up.

Imagine that this light is waking up every part of the body it travels to, invigorating all of the different types of immune cells being made by, and circulating in, your body right now. In the bone marrow, in the glands and nodes, this light is calling upon all your protective cells to function at their highest capacity right now.

Acknowledge that every cell which assists with immunity is receiving the message and beginning to circulate and search for any unusual activity. With a calm alertness, these cells are circulating and looking for foreign cells, or for anything that is harmful or out of place. Your guardian cells are always looking out for you, and their intelligence and sensitivity to even slight differences, fluctuations, or foreign bodies are rapidly increasing. They're becoming more and more specialized— more thorough and better at their jobs every single time they journey through the body.

Imagine your army of immune system cells becoming stronger now and the number of fighters increasing steadily. Your devoted attention is fueling their training and expansion. Keep watching them as they do their work—seeking out invaders and destroying them completely.

Feel your entire body now and imagine it is made up of only healthy, friendly cells. Zoom your attention in onto one singular cell and try to see its shape, brightness, and vibrancy. Notice its capacity to direct change for the better and to produce the most radiant and abundant health possible.

Now begin to see every other cell in the body as replicates of this perfect, clean cell. Billions and trillions of cells, full of white, glowing light and working together harmoniously now. Use the power of your imagination. Let this warm glow flood over the entire body.

Let this glow extend out to the skin and beyond—if you wish, into the space right around your body.

Really try to enjoy this healing sensation that you're creating within and around you. Let the sensation of gratitude, faith, and inner trust live in your awareness. And know that its effects will stay with you long after this meditation ends.

And then, very slowly, shift your attention back to the breath once more. Feel it moving the chest and the tummy up and down—going in and out like gentle, rocking ocean waves.

Notice the body again resting in its seat or lying down, and feel the points of pressure. The weight of the bones. The sensations of the skin and face.

Then, ever so slowly, open your eyes and bring your awareness back into the room.

To the best of your ability, remain present with this new state of healthy awareness as it settles into the physical and mental bodies throughout the next day and night.

Boost your immunity
Studies show that meditation can increase immune health by boosting levels of circulating antibodies, multiplying immune cell count, increasing the lifespan of cells, and having huge anti-inflammatory effects. Indeed, regular practice seems to activate distinct areas of the brain that govern the expression and performance of the immune system.

24

Releasing Negativity

This exercise is meant to help release persistent negative thoughts or patterns, and to assist with mild states of depression—all of which can be normal and natural mental fluctuations as we process more challenging aspects of life such as grief or loss.

One-part meditation

Takes 15–20 minutes

Level Beginner

Preparation Lie on your back and make yourself as comfortable as possible. Let the legs simply fall open to the side, as the hips relax, and tuck the shoulder blades slightly under the back, so the arms are open, with the palms facing up. Make sure the neck is soft and lengthened, using a pillow for support if you wish.

Start to bring your attention to the breath now. Slowly and gradually deepening the breath, slowing it down little by little. Make the inhales and exhales an equal length—effortless and natural. Meanwhile, continue letting the muscles release and sink down, seeing any tension drain away now.

Imagine you can see the sky above you—a pristine, clear blue sky, with a radiant shining sun. Now picture yourself inhaling that luminescent quality directly from the sky, inviting it directly into the body and mind. As it enters the body you can see it feeding and nourishing each and every cell. This energy spreads light and healing automatically—pushing the old, stagnant, or darker qualities residing in our being down farther and farther toward the feet, with every single breath. The inhale receives the luminescent energy gracefully, and the exhale moves all the darkness and heaviness downward and out of the body now.

Observe that with each and every inhale the old, stagnant thoughts held throughout the body are being replaced with bright, healing light. Keep watching this process intently until all of the darkness has exited through the soles of the feet, and is being returned to the Earth to be recycled and re-envisioned.

Now the body is completely made up of glowing, sparkling, positive energy. Notice how this feels. Allow yourself to enjoy the sensation fully. Notice how your thoughts may have shifted or any subtle differences in the physical body.

Take a few moments to continue being still and to bask in this healing light. Become absorbed by it. Let yourself enjoy this inner purification.

You always have the power to return to this state at will, to do more internal healing. With each and every new breath, visualize the cleansing and purifying action. Continue to relax for as long as you like. When you feel ready, softly open your eyes. Begin to move the body, take a couple of deep breaths, and keep this feeling for as long as you can today.

Counteract negativity

Meditation seems to curb negative thoughts and helps bring better-feeling emotional states. It can temper emotional reactivity and also reduce rumination and worry. Meditation also helps us to access the self-referential areas of the brain, allowing us to begin to modify internal stories and reference points that construct sadness and pain.

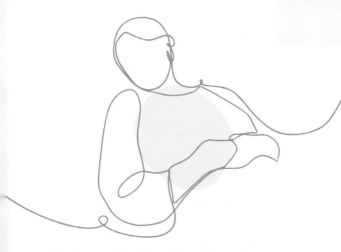

25

Freeing Sadness & Grief

This exercise aims to release negative emotions (such as grief, heartbreak, and other emotional pain), especially when they have been pushed down, remain unexpressed, or have otherwise been stored somewhere in the body. It's widely accepted that unresolved emotion can get trapped in the body and create widely varying levels of physical pain and disease. This practice is one way to assist you in finding and addressing any sorrowfulness that you've experienced enough of and are ready to let go of once and for all.

One-part meditation

Takes 15–20 minutes

Level Beginner

Preparation Find a comfortable position, whether this is lying on your back or seated with a straight spine in a chair or on a cushion on the floor.

Begin by taking some slow, deep breaths and imagine allowing any physical resistance or pain to drain down to the feet and out of the body on each exhale. Breathe in this way, visualizing the muscles releasing more and more until the body feels as soft as possible.

Now bring your awareness down to your feet and begin to scan the body with your attention, slowly moving up and viewing each part until you reach the top of the head. Imagine your attention is like a spotlight and that any discomfort, tension, pain, restriction, grayness, or stagnancy becomes visible under this light. As you slowly make your way up the body, try to notice any areas that may be affected by negativity without engaging with them— without becoming involved in why they are there, how long they've been there, or with any story surrounding the discomfort.

Just simply notice them without judging. As you travel upward with your attention, gently make a mental map of where you notice any gripping or resistance.

When you reach the top of the head, rest your awareness on the sensation of the breath. Feel the movement of the breath in the chest and the belly without trying to change anything about it. Notice its journey in and back out again. Feel the physical body settle more with each exhale, if it needs to.

Now imagine an immensely powerful natural energy—it could be the radiance of sunshine, the purifying power of a waterfall, or the crashing of ocean waves. It could be the dewy mist on a forest floor early in the morning, the iridescent glow of the moon and stars, or anything else that seems appropriate. Visualize a powerful natural charge that feels fresh, pure, and healing for you, coming straight to you from the Earth and the Solar System to support you.

Imagine that energy steadily flowing toward you now and entering your body through the top of your head. See this energy traveling down into any places of discomfort, any places that feel tense or sad or gray. Any spots that feel locked or shut down or depleted.

See this charging energy flooding your system and flushing out any darkness and negativity, leaving in its place just pure, clean, new energy—full of positive potential. Visualize this process as if it is happening right in this moment, directed by your attention.

Your body, mind, and spirit know exactly how to release negative thoughts and rumination, fear and distrust, and other memories and feelings that become harmful when they imbed themselves. Trust in your own wisdom to release what you don't need and witness the action taking place now—simply.

Feel this eternal, life-giving energy filling your system and lighting up everything, all the way out to your skin and even beyond the boundaries of the physical body.

For a few moments continue basking in this new glow. When this exercise ends, you will be carrying the essence of this natural charge in every cell. And your body, mind, and emotions will be transforming under its always-present guidance.

When you feel ready, just begin to feel the body on your support or in your seat. Sense the weight of the body, its posture and shape. Feel the skin and face again. Then very slowly open your eyes and come back into the room. Take a moment to notice how you feel. Smile slightly or breathe a little sigh of relief. Hang onto this feeling as you continue your day with this new, updated version of yourself.

26

Wake Up with Confidence

Early in the morning, before any external stimulation influences your mind, affirm your day. This meditation can help you begin the day with an extra boost of confidence and self-assuredness, so that you can accomplish whatever you set your mind to.

One-part meditation

Takes 10–15 minutes

Level Beginner

Preparation Do this exercise in bed as soon as you wake up in the morning. Roll onto your back, with as little movement as possible, and make yourself comfortable. Without following any thoughts, begin the meditation immediately.

Good morning.

As you slowly begin to bring your awareness from your sleep-state back into the physical space, allow your eyes to stay softly closed and gently direct your thoughts to the sensations present in the physical body now. Bring your attention to the parts of the body where you feel the most pressure against the pillows or bed, and just notice these points of contact. See if you can notice these areas one by one—maybe the heels... the back of the calves... the hips... the rib cage—all of the places where you feel the most contact with your support. Now notice all of these contact areas at the same time. Feel the shape and weight of your entire body now, and notice any physical sensations that are present, without judging. Keep noticing how the body feels right now as you transition from sleep to wakefulness.

Now bring your attention to your breath. Notice the way the breath is moving. After a deep sleep, how does the breath move? How does it act? What can you notice about the quality of your breath right now, as you awaken? Start to breathe in a little bit deeper, inhaling through the nose and exhaling through the nose. Bringing your in- and out-breaths to an equal length. Allowing and watching as the belly and chest rise and fall again.

Imagine you're pulling in lots of extra energy with the air you're inhaling. Imagine this energy as a bright light or a radiant golden color. See it flowing in on the breath and pouring into every corner of the body, naturally seeking out any area that requires energy and support. All by itself the energy is moving in on the breath and touching every important part—you don't have to consciously direct it now. Just inhale and draw a strong breath full of energy, and, as you exhale, it will travel through the body on its own—nourishing and recharging, boosting all the cells, tissues, organs, and more. Enjoy the sensations that appear as this recharging is taking place.

Now imagine the light or color you're inhaling really filling you up—the entire shape of the body, inside the skin. Filling you up not only with energy, but with confidence in particular, and the drive and motivation to move forward toward your goals and dreams. Feel this self-confidence and self-esteem become a new attitude that you're adopting for the day. See it expanding up into the brain and filling the

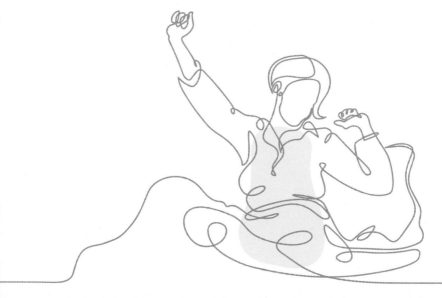

entire skull with light. It's sinking deep into all the regions of the brain and aligning the mind with intention—preparing you for a productive day.

Still focused on this golden energy feeding the body and brain, imagine something that you would love to create or accomplish today. Just one thing. It could be something that must be done, or something that you want to get done. It may be a work-related task or some creative endeavor that you've been wanting to begin or finish. Whatever it is today, bring it to mind.

Place a picture of your goal firmly in your imagination and then see all of this energy effortlessly guiding you toward it. See yourself easily undertaking all of the necessary steps to complete this task or to begin this journey—and, in your mind's eye, try to see yourself actually completing your goal—in as much detail as possible. Try to enjoy that sensation. Really let the feeling of this accomplishment, the feeling of motivation, pride, respect... sink into all of your being. Enjoy the sensation as if it had already happened. Just for a moment, right here and right now.

When this process feels complete for you, bring your awareness fully back to the breath. Start to make small movements... stretching, wiggling the fingers and toes, breathing a little deeper... Preserve this great sensation that you've created in both your mind and body. This air of confidence. The feeling that anything is possible today.

Have a beautiful day.

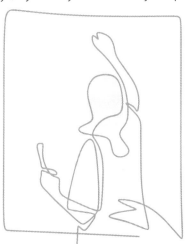

Boost self-esteem
To help you recall a realistic feeling of "confidence," try to remember a time when you did or accomplished something you were very proud of. Recall any praise you may have gotten from others, any acknowledgments. Big or small, this should be something that made you feel good deep down to your core. Now translate that emotional feeling-state to your new visualization for the day.

27

Wake Up to Radiant Health

The first few minutes that we awaken out of a dream-state or a deep sleep, we are very, very receptive to influences and ideas, especially to the auto-suggestion of our own voice and imagination. This meditation can help you visualize entering and beginning your new day in the healthiest, most vibrant state possible.

One-part meditation

Takes 10–15 minutes

Level Beginner

Preparation Do this exercise in bed as soon as you wake up in the morning. Roll onto your back, with as little movement as possible, and make yourself comfortable. Without following any thoughts, begin the meditation immediately.

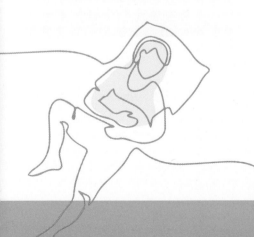

Good morning.

As you gradually come back into an awareness of the physical body, in this physical realm, begin by taking a few moments to just rest in this softness. As you begin to gently bring your attention to the feeling of your physical body again, and the feeling of the breath moving, rising and falling softly at the heart center. Watch the breath fill the space around the heart and channel a sense of self-compassion.

Become aware if there's anything that you would like to shift or facilitate with your own health right now. Is there any place that needs healing or assistance in the physical body? Anywhere in the bones, in the glands, the organs? In the muscles, nerves, tendons, ligaments? The skin, the blood, the blood vessels?

If you recall anything that's ailing you or challenging you physically, imagine that right now and for the next few moments—it's quickly, spontaneously beginning to heal. Take your time, and see and sense the details of it happening for you. Likewise, if there's anything about your body that you'd like to improve, imagine that happening now on its own.

Get the strong sense that your thoughts are powerful enough to create real change. Trust that every cell has the innate knowledge needed to repair correctly and better itself. Know that under the spotlight of your attention, right now, rejuvenation and deep healing are taking place.

You may feel movement in the area—an energy, tingling, or any other sensation. Or you may visualize that you can see deep within the body, that you can vividly watch the body working, detoxifying, renewing, repairing, and reconstructing. Trust fully that this is happening as you witness it in your imagination, and as you sense it throughout your physical body.

If it helps, imagine a time when this part of your body may have been in perfect health—radiant, alive, strong, flexible— and try to find that same sensation and emotion again here and now. Call forward that feeling of perfect health. Allow your cells and tissues to remember that time and to work now from that blueprint of effortless health.

When this process feels complete for you, start to return your awareness to your breath once more. Notice it at the heart center again and get the strong feeling of gratitude for what has and will continue to take place on your account. Feel the breath deepening and extending throughout the body now—charging and activating everything. Start waking the body up, bit by bit. Gently bring your awareness back into the room and let your eyes open.

Have a beautiful day.

Imagine feeling healthy

Every cell holds memory. When we choose to focus our fullest attention on those happy, healthy physical sensations before we had pain or dysfunction, we start to call in more of the same—preparing ourselves to have more joyful embodied experiences. If you've never been without physical discomfort, then try to imagine what it might feel like to wake up in a new body—how would it free you in your mind, your body, and daily activities, your relationships, or in fulfilling your passions? Dive in with your imagination, try to discover the feeling, and use it to focus now.

28

Calming Color Therapy

In this meditation, you'll use a powerful tool of the subconscious—color—to increase the power of visualization and self-healing. You can choose any color that is calming to you for this exercise (people often use lavenders, soft blues, iridescent whites, or warm golden yellows, but any color that comforts you will work). You'll use the power of your imagination to expand this color into every inch of your body—envisioning that wherever the color touches, deep relaxation and healing are taking place automatically.

One-part meditation

Takes 10–15 minutes

Level Beginner to Intermediate

Preparation Find a comfortable position, whether this is lying on your back or seated with a long, straight spine in a chair or on a cushion on the floor.

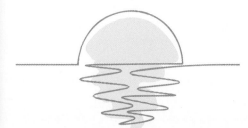

Allow any tension in the body to begin to soften and let your eyes close gently. Find yourself with your breath, moving your attention in and out, as if you were sailing on the breath. Gradually begin to lengthen the breath now. Make the inhales and the exhales an equal length. Keep breathing like this until you feel a subtle sense of calmness wash over you.

Now imagine a color that brings a feeling of calm and peace to you. It could be any color—light blue, lavender, or any color that you find soothing. Take a moment and find the right color for you, right now.

Now imagine that you are breathing in this color as you're inhaling. Bright and dense, this calming color is flowing into your body on every breath in. Inhale, fill your interior with this soothing color. Build the density of this relaxing hue inside the body. Depositing this color throughout. Inhaling, drawing in the color, and exhaling just the breath back out. Inhaling the color, filling from corner to corner of the physical body, and exhaling just the breath back out.

Continue repeating this visualization until the entire shape of the body contains this healing color. Try to feel it saturate your being and bring a sense of serenity to each and every cell. To all of your muscles and bones. All of your organs. Everything... from your skin, inward. Stay here until everything is tinted with serenity.

Now imagine you can breathe through every single pore of your skin at the same time. And begin to inhale through all of the skin, and exhale out the same way, through every inch of the skin. Continue like this, and during the exhale allow anything that feels a bit negative, fearful, anxious, sad, or uneasy that may have been pushed to the outermost corners to simply leave the body and dissipate. Again, inhale the color in through all of the skin, and exhale out anything you no longer need. Repeat until only that pure, calm color exists within you.

When this feels complete, gently guide your attention back to the rising and falling of the chest. The heart center. The natural breath. Watching and observing it wandering in and out of the body, assisting you in every moment with your most crucial plans for growth and healing.

Take a moment to notice how the body, mind, and emotions feel right now.

Begin to notice your body in the room once again. When you're ready, allow your eyes to float open softly and take a moment to enjoy this feeling. With gratitude, acknowledge the time you've taken for yourself.

The more you practice this exercise, the more you can assume conscious control of your own mood and your health.

The power of color
Colors have been used for thousands of years to represent the natural elements, as well as different energy channels and centers in and around the human body. Scientific studies of color therapy show that particular colors encourage the release of neurochemicals, which trigger certain emotions and can affect the nervous system as a whole—stimulating, calming, balancing, and creating healing in the body.

29

Accessing Your Inner Genius

This is a meditation to help you get to know your own inner genius better. In ancient times, it was thought that each person had their own "genius," a guardian spirit of the creative forces that accompanied them throughout life. Everyone's genius is unique, and there are many ways to express your individual inspirations. In fact, your inner genius may inform the way that you do things more than you actually do.

One-part meditation

Takes 10–15 minutes

Level Beginner to Intermediate

Preparation Find any comfortable seated position on a chair or a cushion on the floor where the spine and chest can be lifted, or lie on your back.

Start by relaxing your body as much as you can. Let the tension drain out of your muscles as you breathe in... and out, increasingly calmly and slowly. Feel your body becoming softer and softer on each and every exhale.

Now start to notice your breath. How does it feel right now? Is it deep or shallow? Cool or warm? Try not to change the breath at all—let it be natural and just notice how it feels. And where it's moving in your body. Keep your attention one-pointed on the air going in and coming back out. Imagine you are following it the whole way in, and following it the whole way back out. Is it easy to follow it? Does your attention wander elsewhere? Just notice. Only observing.

Now move your attention to the back of the forehead. Imagine there is a movie screen there behind your eyes and that you can see a beautiful genie's lamp sitting there, just behind your eyes. Notice all of its details. What color is it? What size is it? What shape?

This magical lamp is the container inside you that holds your inner genius. You only have to coax it out.

Now that you can clearly visualize your lamp, let it remain there and turn your mind to something that you really, really love to do. Something you feel good at. Something that comes easily to you. It doesn't matter what it is. Genius inspiration comes in *all* forms. Hint: It's probably something that makes you feel happy and light when you think of it. You would probably say that you feel most like yourself when you're doing this activity...

Try to imagine yourself doing this thing in as much detail as you can possibly visualize—and see how your body reacts. You'll know you've found it when you can use all your senses to imagine it easily and it feels as if it were happening right now.

There may be more than one thing that makes you feel like this—and that's perfectly fine. It's possible you don't know of anything yet that makes you feel this way—and that's also fine. Just continue to focus your attention inward and explore how you feel when you imagine doing the things you love.

Try not to become frustrated if it isn't making sense just yet. Instead, see if you can cultivate a sense of curiosity—even excitement—about what you're going to find inside.

When you think you've found something that expresses your inner passions and gifts, imagine your lamp again. Watch your inner genius materialize from inside the lamp, ready to grant your wish of expressing your desires every day by doing the things that you love—by expressing your unique genius. This force is ready and willing to guide you to reach your fullest potential.

The spirit of your unique gifts is always waiting inside for you to seek its guidance. It is eternally channeling inspiration to you in the form of the dreams, insights, and passions that most excite you in this life.

When you feel ready, start to notice your breath again. See it moving naturally in and out... Rising and falling. Follow it for a few moments.

Now feel your body begin to energize a bit more, with every inhale—re-engaging with the physical body and the physical space it's in—then slowly open your eyes.

Return to this meditation regularly to enhance your concentration and to get closer to your inner genius and the cultivation of your life's passion.

30

Yoga Nidra Deep Healing Relaxation

In yoga nidra, or "psychic sleep," the practitioner accesses a state between wakefulness and sleep by listening to the guided meditation while keeping still. It is crucial you do not move, even an inch, during this practice. You are aiming to lose all bodily sensation, so your awareness is fully directed inward. The physical, mental, and energetic bodies relax, and the subconscious gets a chance to redirect vital life force to any place that most needs healing— directed by your inner knowing and intentional key phrase.

One-part meditation

Takes 25–45 minutes

Level Beginner to Intermediate

Preparation Lie on your back in bed or on the floor/a mat. Use pillows and blankets to make yourself comfortable, so you won't have to move—a pillow under the knees will relax the lower spine. Use a phrase to act as a seed for your subconscious, something short that focuses on your own inner healing. Try: "My concentration is increasing rapidly"; "I am now accessing my inner guidance"; or "I now easily move toward my innermost passions." You'll repeat this phrase during the deepest part of the relaxation as an autosuggestion. Try to use the same one each time you practice, as the benefits are cumulative.

See the muscles softening. Let everything begin melting down and allow the body to slip into deep relaxation. Notice how even the breath is slowing down, all by itself.

Bring your awareness to the left foot. With your attention strongly engaged, ask the toes to relax, one by one. See each toe soften and release. See the left foot— both the sole and the top of the foot. Place all your attention there, flooding the area and everything in between. Relax the left foot. All fatigue and tension melting out. Bring your focus now to the left ankle. Relax the ankle, all the way through, letting go of any discomfort or sensations.

Now move to the left lower leg and calf. Muscles melting away from the bone, totally relaxed. Move now to the left knee. From front to back, and to each side, and all the way through the joint, see every structure softening and warming. Relax. Move on to the left upper leg and thigh now. Feel it becoming heavier, softening down—release. The left hip—all the way around to the seat. Everything warming, sinking down heavy. Relax even more now.

Now move your attention down to the right foot and toes. Begin by relaxing the toes, one by one. Softening, warming, releasing. Relax the sole and the top of the foot, and everything in between. Moving the attention to the right ankle, seeing everything there let go. The right lower leg and calf, warming and melting. Release all tension. Now to the right knee, all the way through, seeing lots of space to release inside. The right thigh and upper leg—the muscles, nerves, bones—sinking down heavy. Release. The right hip, all the way through to the seat—everything melting down. Soft and heavy.

Move now to the lower back and spine. Visualize lots of space between the vertebrae—muscles and nerves relaxing away from the bones. Warm and heavy. Release the lower back. The middle back and spine now. Allow it to feel spacious and free. Broadening and sinking down—very heavy. Relax. The upper back, spine, and shoulder blades. All layers releasing, one by one. Heaving down, tension draining away. Relax.

Bring your attention to the abdomen. See it warming, softening, sinking down. The solar plexus area—surrendering, giving

way to warm, gentle sensation. The chest and rib cage—soft, light, and free. Feel a sense of openness as the muscles of the front body relax down and back.

Now move your attention to the left hand and fingertips. Relax the fingers, letting them unfold and soften down, with the palm melting open. No more sense of grasping. Just the freedom of letting go. The left forearm—all the muscles melting away. Dissolving. The left elbow and upper arm—heavy, sinking away from the body. Relax. Now the right hand and fingertips. Melting open, soft and loose. Release the right forearm now—muscles melting away from bone. The right elbow and upper arm—sinking down, tension disappearing.

Both shoulders rolling back now and sinking down deeply. Release. The neck and throat—all tension draining away. Feel the entire area warm and supple, melting down further.

Soften the jaw, the area around the mouth, cheeks, and nose, and relax the area around the eyes and temples. Let the forehead and scalp warm and melt back even further now. Relax.

See the internal organs resting now. Peacefully sinking back. Imagine everything is working perfectly. Relax here.

Now imagine your body is getting very heavy. Extremely heavy. Sinking down into and through the support—as if the body was made of lead. Imagine with all of your senses. See the body getting extremely heavy. Feel gravity pulling it down.

Now imagine your body is becoming lighter—very light. And even beginning to float upward... floating up several inches off the support. The body is extremely light now, like a feather. Feel this effervescent feeling in every part of the body, as it continues to get lighter and lighter.

Now imagine your body is getting very cold. Imagine yourself lying underneath snow—with ice all around you—feeling extremely cold. Chilled to the bone. Very, very cold. Remember what this feels like.

Imagine now that your body is becoming warmer—getting hot. Imagine yourself in the desert, in the midday sun. Very, very hot now. Hot sand beneath your feet, hot sun on your skin, and sweat coming from every pore. Extremely hot.

Now imagine you're a perfect temperature. Extremely comfortable. Lying in the grass, on a hillside. Soft earth and green grass supporting you. The air is the perfect temperature for you, with a gentle breeze in the nearby trees. Crystal blue skies above with an occasional soft, white cloud floating by. Beautiful trees and flowers nearby. Everything is perfectly comfortable. There's nowhere to go, nothing to do. All sense of time releases.

All sense of urgency releases. Birds sing in a nearby tree. And you hear the sound of tranquil water in the distance.

Allow yourself to rest here—completely. Enjoying with all of your senses. Smelling the scents, seeing the colors, hearing the sounds. Allow the body to rest back, perfectly supported by the Earth. Relax.

Now place your attention either at the center of your chest or the back of the forehead, and focus your consciousness there. Now repeat the intention you created, repeating it to yourself three times, with faith. Rest for a while longer now, remaining unconcerned. Very, very slowly... start to notice your breath again, rising and falling in the body, moving all by itself. Notice the feeling of the air on your skin and face, and your body in the room.

Begin to move and stretch the physical body, as if you were just waking out of a deep sleep. Little by little, moving however feels right to you, right now. Eventually, bring yourself up to sit, or continue to rest on your back with your awareness re-engaged. Take a few moments to notice just how you feel.

Meditation Directory

Use this directory if you have a specific issue you would like to address or a desired meditative effect that you'd like to achieve. Depending on your goal, it will direct you to a guided meditation or section in the book with meditations that can help. You can search through some common physical conditions that are often helped with meditation.

Anxiety and Stress Reduction

When worry, fear, or rumination become persistent they can affect all aspects of life and our relationships, making even simple everyday tasks seem insurmountable. Anxiety can be a normal response in novel or challenging situations, but when the neural pathways that activate anxious behavior stay engaged longer than they should, then even small tasks and daily functioning can be affected.

Chapter 1/Mindful (pages 16–57)
Chapter 2/Calm (pages 58–91)
Dissolve Mental Stress (page 98)
Calming Color Therapy (page 115)
Yoga Nidra Deep Healing Relaxation (page 119)

Chronic Pain

Chronic pain is produced less by actual tissue damage and more by active neural patterns related to previous injury, perceived damage and disability, and fear. Meditation can help reduce the perception of pain by instilling a sense of control over one's own health. Some exercises that can help to ease the burden of chronic pain include:

Body Scan (page 20)
Mindful Awareness of the Breath (page 26)
Mindful Awareness of Sounds (page 32)
Mindful Awareness of Thoughts (page 38)
Calming Breath (page 62)
Breathing for Physical Release (page 70)
Progressive Muscle Relaxation (page 72)
Affirming Serenity (page 75)
Wake Up to Radiant Health (page 113)
Yoga Nidra Deep Healing Relaxation (page 119)

Note
Meditation has many benefits, but it should not be used as a substitute for professional medical advice or treatment.

Communication

Communication is the basis of all relationships. Society expects us to communicate our own desires and needs, and also hear and respond to those of others (like family, partners, friends, bosses, and coworkers), all while setting and maintaining boundaries or managing expectations. When we skillfully accomplish this, we can create opportunities where none seem to exist and protect ourselves from unnecessary stressful situations that might hijack our energy and lead us off-track.

Chapter 1/Mindful (pages 16–57)
Calming Breath (page 62)
Stress Reduction SSS-Breath (page 68)
Affirming Serenity (page 75)
Wake Up with Confidence (page 110)

Creativity

Creative thinking and problem-solving is ignited when we are able to access, recruit, and integrate more parts of the brain than we would during rote-learning or daily routines. Scientists concur that changing things up and trying things that may feel uncomfortable at first can actually heighten our ability to innovate. Deep relaxation where we can examine the unconscious can stimulate novel, creative output.

Chapter 1/Mindful (pages 16–57)
Energy Boost (page 96)
Dissolve Mental Stress (page 98)
Wake Up with Confidence (page 110)
Accessing Your Inner Genius (page 117)

Depression

Hundreds of millions of people suffer from
sadness, disinterest, or hopelessness on an
ongoing basis. Depression is brought on by an
interplay of psychological, biological, and social
factors. Chronic stress and traumatic events can
fuel depression, and depression can affect
everything, from physical health to relationships
to quality of life.

Chapter 1/Mindful (pages 16–57)
Affirming Serenity (page 75)
Easy Sleep (page 87)
Energy Boost (page 96)
Dissolve Mental Stress (page 98)
Releasing Negativity (page 106)
Freeing Sadness & Grief (page 108)
Wake Up with Confidence (page 110)
Accessing Your Inner Genius (page 117)

Focus/Productivity

In a world made of distractions (expansive social
media, email, pings, and pop-ups, and the internet
in general), most people deal with some degree
of distraction on a daily basis that affects their
thoughts, plans, and tasks. In modern society our
attention is so split and dispersed that deep focus
and engagement on one task at a time is quickly
becoming extinct, even though many studies
show that "multitasking" is ineffective at best. Our
brains are wired to do one task at a time, and
when our attention is split positive outcomes are
greatly diminished.

Chapter 1/Mindful (pages 16–57)
Ocean Breath (page 78)
Energy Boost (page 96)
Dissolve Mental Stress (page 98)
Wake Up with Confidence (page 110)
Accessing Your Inner Genius (page 117)

Headaches

Different types of headaches have different sets of
causes and can produce varying symptoms,
including localized head pain, referred pain, nausea,
vision problems, and a lack of mental focus. Many
symptoms can be eased by practicing meditations
such as these:

Breathing for Physical Release (page 70)
Progressive Muscle Relaxation (page 72)
Dissolve Mental Stress (page 98)
Wake Up to Radiant Health (page 113)
Calming Color Therapy (page 115)

High Blood Pressure

Reducing stress can have an immediately positive effect on hypertension by activating the parasympathetic nervous system, which signals a release of hormones that lowers the pressure in the circulatory system by dilating the vessels, slowing heart rate, and slowing down the breath. Learning to use breathing and meditation exercises on a regular basis can impact the chronic stress that promotes hypertension.

Body Scan (page 20)
Mindful Awareness of the Breath (page 26)
Chapter 2/Calm (pages 58–91)
Dissolve Mental Stress (page 98)
Heart Health (page 100)
Wake Up to Radiant Health (page 113)

Immune System Disorders

The immune system includes glands and nodes, membranes, bone marrow, the skin, and blood cells. It normally provides protection against invaders such as bacteria, viruses, and other foreign bodies. Sometimes the immune system is turned around, seeing the body's healthy, normal cells as a threat and attacking them. Both a diminished immune system (think asthma or eczema) or one that is overactive and destroying familiar cells (think rheumatoid arthritis or MS) can take a toll on the quality of life. Many cancers are also thought to affect or be affected by the immune system.

Body Scan (page 20)
Mindful Awareness of the Breath (page 26)
Mindful Awareness of Sounds (page 32)
Mindful Awareness of Thoughts (page 38)
Mindfulness of Support from the Ground (page 46)
Mindfulness of Compassion (page 50)
Chapter 2/Calm (pages 58–91)
Immunity Boost (page 103)
Yoga Nidra Deep Healing Relaxation (page 119)

Insomnia

About 30 percent of the population report sleep disturbances, which can contribute to lowered immunity, an increased perception of pain, a diminished capacity for decision-making and learning, an increase in inflammation, and more. Try these exercises to retrain your sleep habits:

Progressive Muscle Relaxation (page 72)
Countdown to Sleep (page 85)
Easy Sleep (page 87)
Guided Sleep Relaxation (page 89)
Yoga Nidra Deep Healing Relaxation (page 119)

Nervous System and Brain Health

The nervous system includes the brain, spinal cord, and nerves and nerve cells that act as a complex system of communication—receiving sensory input, directing physical actions (both gross and microscopic), learning and thinking, expressing and feeling emotion, and more. The nervous system governs all aspects of our experience in the world.

Body Scan (page 20)
Mindful Awareness of the Breath (page 26)
Mindful Awareness of Sounds (page 32)
Mindful Awareness of Thoughts (page 38)
Mindfulness of Walking (page 48)
Mindfulness of Compassion (page 50)
Mindful Listening & Communication (page 54)
Calming Breath (page 62)
Stress Reduction SSS-Breath (page 68)
Belly Breathing (page 80)
Guided Sleep Relaxation (page 89)
Wake Up to Radiant Health (page 113)
Calming Color Therapy (page 115)
Yoga Nidra Deep Healing Relaxation (page 119)

PMS

Premenstrual syndrome can affect as many as 90 percent of menstruating women. Its symptoms can be mild or severe and may change or fluctuate throughout a lifetime. Anxiety and irritability, depression, muscle and joint pain, abdominal cramping, fatigue, sensitivity to light and sound, migraines and other headaches, and insomnia are all commonly experienced by women around a week to ten days before their period.

Body Scan (page 20)
Mindful Awareness of the Breath (page 26)
Mindful Awareness of Thoughts (page 38)
Mindfulness of Compassion (page 50)
Chapter 2/Calm (pages 58–91)
Energy Boost (page 96)
Releasing Negativity (page 106)
Wake Up with Confidence (page 110)
Calming Color Therapy (page 115)
Accessing Your Inner Genius (page 117)
Yoga Nidra Deep Healing Relaxation (page 119)

Pregnancy

Pregnancy comes with many physical and emotional challenges. The physical body must expand, adjust, and reposition to accommodate a growing baby, and hormonal surges can alter mood and perception. Additionally, sleep and eating habits are altered, and some self-care habits may be inaccessible for a time. Any meditations that decrease anxiety can be of benefit, including:

Body Scan (page 20)
Mindful Awareness of the Breath (page 26)
Breathing for Physical Release (page 70)
Progressive Muscle Relaxation (page 72)
Affirming Serenity (page 75)
Countdown to Sleep (page 85)
Guided Sleep Relaxation (page 89)
Wake Up to Radiant Health (page 113)
Calming Color Therapy (page 115)

Index

A
acceptance 25
ailments, physical 70, 72
anxiety 122

B
benefits, of meditation 12, 102
body scan exercises 20–25,
    46–47
brain health 126
brain networks 18
breath/breathing 14, 26–31
    as an anchor 31
    belly 80–84
    calming 62–67
    controlling 84
    counting 63–64, 66, 73
    healing 71
    mindfulness 26–31
    ocean 78–79
    physical release 70–71
    slowing the 60, 84
    stress reduction sss- 68–69
    tips for 67
    yoga 78–79

C
calm 60–91
chakras 14
children 13
chronic pain 122
color therapy 115–116
communication 54–57, 123
compassion 50–53
confidence 110–112
counting 62–64, 66–67, 73, 78,
    81–82, 85–86, 101–102
creativity 123

D
depression 106, 124
dialogues, internal 13, 54–55,
    75–77

diaphragm 80–84

E
eating 44–45
energy boost 96–97
everyday-life moments 49, 57

F
focus/productivity 124
food 44–45

G
genius, accessing your inner
    117–118
grief, freeing 108–109

H
headaches 98–99, 124
healing breath 71
heart health 100–102
high blood pressure 125

I
immune system 103–105, 125
insomnia 125

L
listening 54–57, 123

M
meditation journey, starting the
    12–13
mindfulness meditations 18–57
muscles 14–15, 72–74

N
negativity, releasing 106–107
nervous system 60, 87, 126
nidra deep healing relaxation, yoga
    119–121

O
ocean breath 78–79

P
phrases, repeating 52–53, 76–77,
    88
PMS (premenstrual syndrome)
    126
pregnancy 126
preparation 14–15
productivity/focus 124
progressive muscle relaxation
    (PMR) 72–74

R
reflective listening 56–57
resistance 51, 77, 88, 94–95,
    108–9

S
sadness, freeing 108–109
scene, changing the 37
self-esteem, boosting 112
serenity, affirming 75–77
sleep 85–91
sounds 32–37
spine 14
stress 60, 68–69, 72, 98–99, 122

T
thought patterns 43
thoughts 38–43
tips, starting 15

V
visualization exercises 60, 69–70,
    91, 96–121
visualization practice 94–95, 99

W
waking up 110–114
walking 48–49
wellbeing, source of 53

Y
yoga 78–79, 119–121

Acknowledgments

Eternal thanks to my mother and father for their constant, unconditional support.

Thank you to all of my past, current, and future teachers and mentors who have helped me in so many ways to gain self-knowledge and the skills to assist other people.

Special thanks to Sri Dharma Mittra, for being an example of pristine spirit and humbleness on my path.

Thanks to Rachel Beider for believing in me and sharing opportunities for growth.

Thank you to my close support network of friends who continue to believe in me as I grow and evolve in this life.

And thank you to the team at Quarto for being so helpful and gracious.

Picture Credits
Andyfirm/Shutterstock.com; Askhat Gilyakhov/Shutterstock.com; Back one line/Shutterstock.com; Derplan13/Shutterstock.com; DODOMO/Shutterstock.com; Kamila Bay/Shutterstock.com; karakotsya/Shutterstock.com; LivDeco/Shutterstock.com; LuckyStep/Shutterstock.com; Magic Panda/Shutterstock.com; Marchrushka/Shutterstock.com; Mikhail Gnatuyk/Shutterstock.com; NikVector/Shutterstock.com; one line man/Shutterstock.com; pimchawee/Shutterstock.com; Singleline/Shutterstock.com; Retany/Shutterstock.com; Valenty/Shutterstock.com

Recorded Guided Meditations
If you wish to record some meditations from this book as audio practices, the free downloads at the following link will give you an idea of the pace and tone that is often used: www.cntrdwellness.com/audio-meditations